The Miracle of Baby J

Jenessa's Journey

By:
Debbie Sherman

PublishAmerica
Baltimore

First printing

Some pictures are courtesy of www.skstone.com

ISBN: 1-59286-740-5
PUBLISHED BY PUBLISHAMERICA, LLLP
www.publishamerica.com
Baltimore

Printed in the United States of America

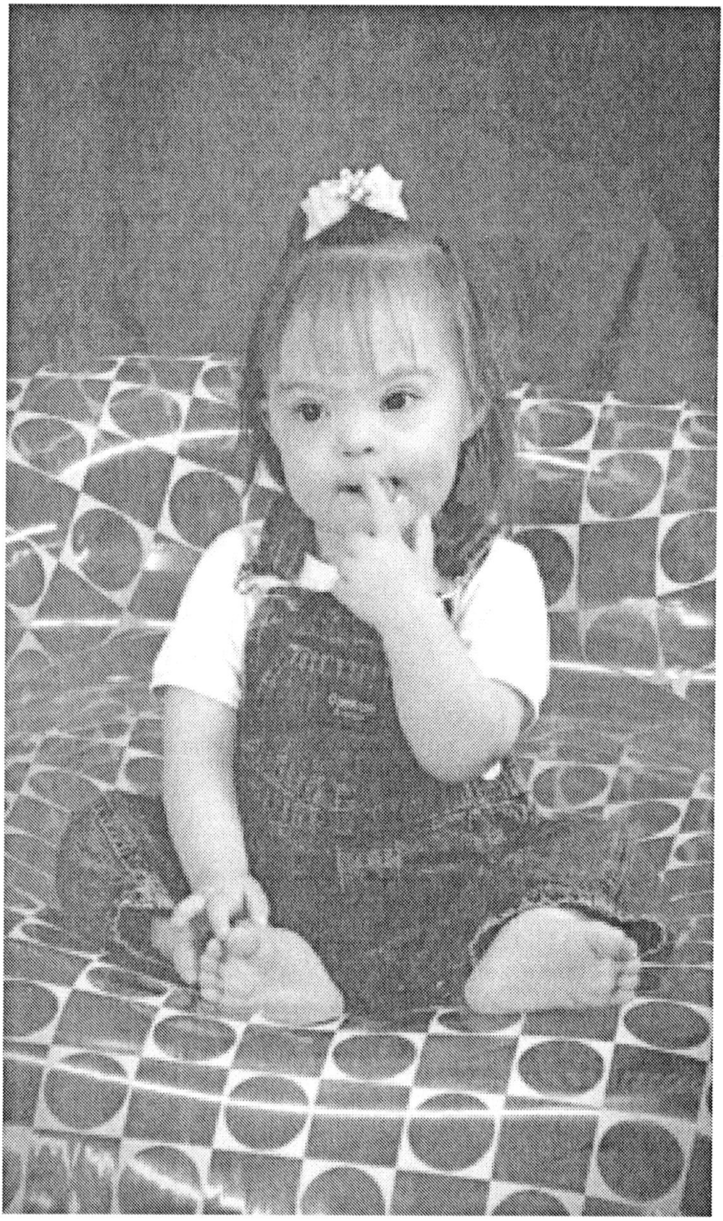

Jenessa's Journey

Song Lyrics

Written by Jackie Bermingham, age 15
(Jenessa's Sister)

Chorus:
I know it was supposed to be her
I know it was meant to be
I know she was the perfect addition to our family.

Have you ever seen a miracle happen?
Do you watch one every day?
The story of Jenessa's Journey is what I'm trying to portray…

She was tiny and not too stable
With the tears and a heart defect
The surgeries and the pain I can easily recollect…

Chorus
I know it was supposed to be her
I know it was meant to be
I know she was the perfect addition to our family.

The days and the nights in the hospital
Were more than just a few,
God her first weeks alive were spent in there with You.

Holding her in my arms
Was like there was an angel there,
I held her hands and rubbed my fingers
Through her abundance of hair.

Chorus:
I know it was supposed to be her
I know it was meant to be
I know she was the perfect addition to our family.

The tubes they stuck in,
The blood they took out,
Was more than enough to make you shout!

Then the day came
When we brought her home,
Where she belonged with us all along.

Chorus:
I know it was supposed to be her
I know it was meant to be
I know she was the perfect addition to our family.

As we fast-forward to today
I watch her walk and talk with a smile,
Knowing God stood by her side all the while.

Lord, I thank you for my sister Jenessa,
Who I love with all my heart,
Who was destined to be with us from the very start.

Lord you knew you were gonna send her to us,
You knew it was meant to be,
You knew she was the perfect addition to our family…

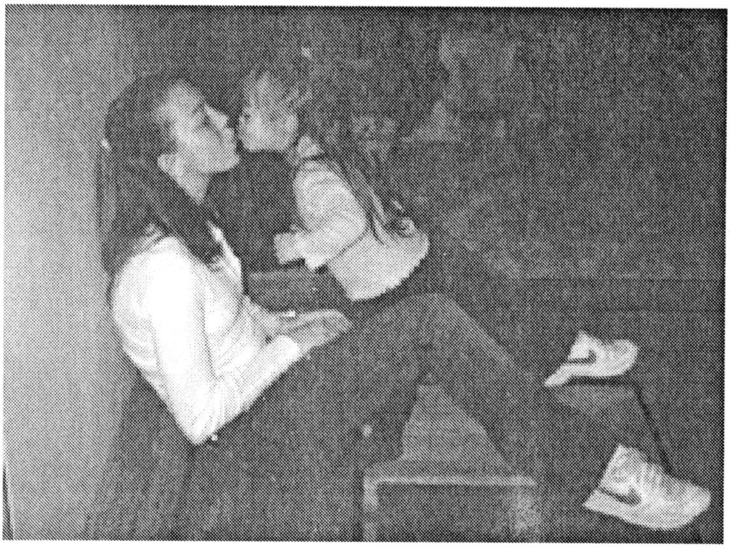

With God, all things are possible.

Acknowledgements:

First and foremost I need to thank my husband Bill, for never doubting Jenessa should be brought into this world. Thank you for helping me conceive our beautiful daughter.

Special thanks to Justin, Jackie, and Jessi, for loving their sister with a deep and profound love, and for opening their hearts to experience the joy that Jenessa brings to their lives.

Heartfelt thanks to Dr. Douglas King, Georgia Ditzenberger, Dr. Jim Croom, and Dr. Lawrence Leichtman, for your brilliant contributions to this book. I am so very grateful for the time and effort you so generously gave to this project.

Thanks also to my mother, for allowing her pre-conceived notions about Down syndrome to be redefined. To Bill's parents, for loving their granddaughter completely and without hesitation.

Thank you to all the brilliant doctors, nurses, and EMT's who have played a part in Jenessa's care. Especially to Dr. Douglas King, Georgia Ditzenberger, Dr. Cynthia Cristofani, Jennie Peterson, Maureen Jones, Dr. John Iguidbashian, Dr. Albert Starr, Dr. Carolyn Merten, and Chris Dugan. Thanks also to everyone in the PICU at Legacy Emanuel Children's Hospital, and the NICU at Doernbecher Children's Hospital. Your time, knowledge, and incredible dedication are unparalleled.

A very special thank you to Margo Dueber. You have been such an anchor of support for me; a great friend and amazing shoulder to lean on. Not only were you there throughout my pregnancy and those first scary months, but still now, you are such a bright spot in my life. Your love and humor have been such a gift. Thank you for encouraging me to write this book, and for listening and watching as Jenessa's Journey took on a life of it's own. (Of course it did!!)

Special thanks to all my incredible friends, especially Denise Hippensteel, and Debbie Kennedy. I don't know what I would do without you. Your constant love and encouragement have meant more to me than mere words could possibly convey. You are truly God's angels, and I'm grateful He sent you into my life.

Thank you to *everyone* at Seaside Christian Church, for all your love, prayers, and support. Especially to Betty Westhoven, for heading up the prayer chain and making sure that Jenessa was constantly in everyone's hearts and prayers. To Pastors Michael Hague and Terry O'Casey, for being available whenever we needed you. Thank you for holding our hands.

Thanks also to Dr. Deborah Cahill and Dr. Carey Winkler, for providing me (and Jenessa!) with the very best of pre-natal care.

Thank you to Laurie Kyllo, for asking me to speak to her class of nursing students during their pediatric study unit. It was overwhelming for me to watch Jenessa's story have such an impact on the way those students will someday practice medicine.

Thank you also to Dan Anderson and Emily Perl Kingsley, for allowing me to include their beautiful work in my book.

And to *all* our friends and family who pitched in while I was at the hospital with Jenessa, thank you for giving me the gift of time. And for the peace of mind to know that my children were well taken care of in my absence.

But mostly, I have to thank Him.
With God, all things are possible.

Debbie

Table of CONTENTS

CONTENTS

CONTENTS

CHAPTER ONE:

THE SKY IS FALLING

I remember the sound of the telephone the day my doctor called with the results from my Alpha- fetoprotein (AFP) test. She said the results were 'off', and that she probably had just made a mistake on my due date. She explained that if your due date is calculated incorrectly, and you take an AFP test too early, then the results can come out wrong. She was certain that explained the funny results. Well, maybe. Maybe I should take another AFP test in another week. Without getting too nervous, I agreed to the additional test. You know, just to be sure. After all, I wanted to rule out the possibility that my baby might have Down syndrome, so I could relax and enjoy the rest of my pregnancy. So on May 26, my 39th birthday, I took the blood test, again.

> The alpha-fetoprotein test is also known as the triple screen test. Blood is drawn from the expectant mother between 16-18 weeks of pregnancy. A laboratory then measures the levels of three substances: 1. Alpha-fetoprotein: a protein produced by the liver of the fetus, 2. Estriol: a pregnancy hormone, and 3. Human Chorionic Gonadotropin: another pregnancy hormone. Elevated levels of alpha-fetoprotein can indicate the presence of a neural tube defect, such as, spina bifida or anencephaly, failure of the brain to develop. Low levels of alpha-fetoprotein and estriol, combined with elevated levels of HCG, can indicate Down syndrome. However, abnormal levels in this 'triple screen' test are not by themselves diagnostic. They

merely indicate a risk and that further tests, such as ultrasound or amniocentesis, should be considered.

When I heard from my OBGYN, she was concerned and confused. The results hadn't changed; the count was still 'off'. She still felt everything was probably okay, as these tests were sometimes inconclusive. After all, the baby had a good, strong heartbeat, and her growth rate was in line with her gestational age. But she suggested that I see a specialist, called a perinatalogist. (At that time I didn't even know what this specialist was, let alone how to spell it!) There I could be given one of those new high-tech ultrasounds, where you get a clearer view of the baby. They could do special measurements, and give me an amniocentesis if they thought it was necessary. This way, we could rule out for sure any chromosomal disorders.

Before we even had a chance to digest what all of this might mean, my husband Bill and I were sitting in the perinatalogists office. Only a few days had passed since the results from the first tests; *those* days had been spent wandering around in a fog. Now we were listening as the doctor explained the ultrasound procedure to us, which seemed simple enough. They would look, they would measure, they would calculate. Depending on the findings, they would decide whether or not to proceed with the amniocentesis. Because their equipment was so high-tech, the amnio could be done with the smallest of risks.

The ultrasound was amazing! I could see my baby's tiny face. The fingers, the feet....wow. In past ultrasounds I could barely make out the baby; I always thought the baby looked more like an alien than an actual child. This time I could see the eyes, the nose, the tiny little arms and legs. When the baby rolled over with legs apart, my husband and the doctors assured me we were expecting a girl.

The technicians measured her femur lengths, which are usually shorter in babies with Down syndrome. Hers were normal. Her features looked normal. Her brain measurements were normal. All of her internal organs measured normal. Next they measured her neck, which is usually a big, tell-tale sign. Short, thick necks are commonplace in kids with Down syndrome. Hers was normal. The technicians were all starting to smile, and the tension in the room was easing with each bit of good news. Only one more hurdle: her heart. If this appeared normal too, the doctors felt the amnio wouldn't even be necessary.

In the next five minutes, everything changed. Her heart had a hole between three of its four chambers. One of her arteries was too small, and not enough blood was flowing where it was supposed to flow. Before long, Dr. Douglas King, MD, a specialist in pediatric cardiology, was brought into the room. He began circling the "defects" on the screen. He explained to us what was wrong with our baby's heart. He used a pointer on the screen to show us the specific defects, and explained to us the inner workings of the heart. His first diagnosis was twofold; our baby had Tetralogy of Fallot and a complete Atrioventricular Canal Defect (complete medical details and diagnosis can be found at the end of the book). I had no idea what this man was talking about; I didn't want to understand. I couldn't even make out the heart on the screen, let alone the vessels and chambers. I couldn't listen anymore.

So Bill listened, and Bill understood. I remember thinking *okay–okay*, she has a heart defect. That doesn't mean she has Down syndrome. The doctors felt that because of her AFP results *and* this, we should go ahead with the amnio. We agreed. Results from an amnio generally take about two weeks to get back, but the doctors were aware of a new process that could provide answers within 48 hours. They decided they would have my amniotic fluid sent to this special laboratory, so we wouldn't have to spend the next two weeks worrying.

The amnio itself was mostly uneventful and just a bit uncomfortable, but nothing I couldn't handle. Bill held my hand throughout the procedure, and then, that was it. We were 'excused' and could go home. Just like that. Get dressed and go home, and pretend that this entire appointment had not taken place. Oh, wait. The doctor wanted to discuss our options with us.

If the test did in fact come back positive, meaning that the baby would have Down syndrome, of course, we could choose to keep the baby (how nice to be given that option!). But we needed to *be prepared for the many challenges that a Down child would bring.* He said life as we knew it would no longer exist, and we would need to come to grips with that. I already had three children; life had never been the same after any of them! The doctor went on and on, and explained that in Oregon we had until the 24th week to legally terminate a pregnancy. He suggested we give this some serious thought. Did he really need to say that? Did he think we were just going to go home and *not* think about it!?

Next, Dr. King came back into the room. He explained that if we decided to keep the baby, he would support us fully and be there every step of the way. He impressed upon us the seriousness of her heart defects, and the extreme medical challenges she would face. He would do periodic echo-cardiograms (basically an ultrasound of the heart) through my belly, and keep us posted on the growth her heart made in-utero. My head was spinning. I couldn't speak. Bill and I exchanged glances and thoughts, the way married people do, but said nothing.

As I was dressing and preparing to leave, a nurse came in and gave us a handout on Down syndrome, which I quickly threw into my purse. Somehow I managed to finish dressing, and we left the office without making a scene.

It was a long, quiet, two hour drive home. I decided to read the handout, and it was appalling. It made it sound like the worst possible life any human being could have. I remember getting about halfway through it, with tears running down my face, when I told Bill that I couldn't knowingly bring a child into this world, who would have to live like that. One who is sick all the time and not able to hold her head up, ever. Being mentally retarded, never learning how to do everyday, simple tasks, and never understanding anything of value. It sounded like a cruel existence, without hope. We were horrified.

Once we got home, I talked Bill into going back to work. I called my mother, and told her about my day. She felt that I was too old, and already had too much on my plate to raise a disabled child. After all, I was constantly on the go with Justin, who played on a traveling soccer team. And Jackie, my mother felt, kept me busy enough with basketball and softball, and oh, yeah– we had just adopted Jessi eight months ago. She told me stories about a thrift shop near her home that employed women with Down syndrome.

"They're really sweet", she said. "There's one gal who introduces herself to me every time I shop there, and often more than once during the same visit."

She spoke of these women as meaning well, but slow, and told me how it took them forever to ring up her purchases. Then she told me about an acquaintance of hers who has an older daughter with Down syndrome. Apparently, the girls' father was a wealthy doctor. My mother believed that because price was no object, that child was given every possible advantage. She'd had top specialists and top care, but was still unable to do much of anything for herself. My mom just kept insisting that it would be too much for me to handle at this stage of my life. She did admit, however, that she would understand Bill's desire to have this child, as it would be his first child by birth. (Jackie and Justin are mine from a previous marriage, and Jessi, as you just read, is adopted.) Oh, did she feel sorry for me! She ended by saying that she would stand by whatever decision we made, but it was clear that she felt we should terminate the pregnancy if it turned out that the baby would have Down syndrome.

Next, I went to my computer; being completely ignorant on the subject, I wanted to read everything I could find on Down syndrome. The web sites were endless. I read from medical journals, from medical files, from dictionaries, educational sites, chromosome experts, scientific studies, and more. Everything I read was *positive.* Everything I read said not to read or believe anything that was not written in the past five years. There had been so much work done in this field in recent years; so many scientific breakthroughs and medical advances that have replaced earlier thinking, findings, and expectations. Limits were no longer being placed on kids with Down syndrome. These children were being raised in families, not institutions. They had wonderful and fulfilling lives. They learned. They grew. They were real people who could lead real lives. This was nothing at all like the information printed on the handout from the doctor's office. The handout turned out to be twenty years old, written back when they sent kids with *any* disabilities to institutions. This got me thinking. If you put a perfectly healthy child into an institution instead of into a loving family, how well would that child cope? How well could that child be expected to cope? The environment in which a child is brought up in helps form the child. Therefore, a warm, loving home would be far more conducive to raising a warm, loving child than a medical institution. Even the best institution couldn't provide what a home could. So putting a child with Down syndrome into an institution was about as ridiculous as putting a healthy baby into one. This wasn't rocket science; this was obvious, even to me.

Still surfing on my computer, I read excerpts from books and magazines. I read many inspirational stories, and realized most people did not feel that having a child with Down syndrome was a bad thing. Most people actually spoke of their child as being special or gifted; not in the conventional way, but gifted nonetheless. This way of thinking appealed to me, and touched me in ways I cannot possibly explain. I was really in the dark before this; I didn't know any disabled children. Sure, I'd seen lots of movies, and had usually been moved to tears whenever a disabled child had been involved, but I didn't know any. I'd never really given it much thought. Of course, I knew that any number of things could go wrong during my pregnancy. I was one of those people who said "I don't care if it's a boy or a girl, as long as my baby's healthy." I'd suffered a miscarriage before Justin had been born, and until now, that had been my biggest worry. The thought that my baby might have Down syndrome, or any other syndrome, had never occurred to me before my AFP test. When I first heard of the possibility a few weeks ago, I was terrified. I was angry. I called a friend and asked what had I done wrong in my life that God would punish me in such a way? She insisted that God didn't work that way, but at the time, I hadn't been ready to listen. But as I sat there, in front of my computer, I found myself overwhelmed with a sense of calmness. Reading about these children was uplifting and encouraging, not depressing like I had imagined.

Medically, I learned a lot. I was most comforted when I learned, nothing Bill and/or I had done could have caused this to happen. Down syndrome is the most common of all genetic abnormalities, and happens in the earliest stages of creation, when the cells are dividing and separating. It's usually caused by an error in cell division called non-disjunction. Instead of having 46 chromosomes in your cells, people with Down syndrome have 47. They have an extra portion of the number 21 chromosome present in all, or some, of their cells. This additional genetic material alters the course of development that causes the characteristics associated with Down syndrome. There are hundreds of books and web-sites that explain this in much greater, far more scientific detail, so I'll leave that to the experts.

Next, I stumbled across other peoples' personal stories and testimonies. The only explanation I can give for how and why I stumbled across these stories, is that, I was supposed to. I know that I was meant to read *these* stories on *this* day. They changed my outlook. They changed my life. The very first one I read was about a 7 year old girl. She was really quite cute! Her parents credited her development with 3 things: 1. God, 2. medical science, and 3. TNI. I knew about God. I knew about medical science. I went to a search engine and typed in TNI. Turns out the initials stood for Targeted Nutritional Intervention. It was all about getting kids with Down syndrome the vitamins, minerals, amino acids, anti-oxidants, and other nutrients that they need for better growth, better brain development, a healthier immune system, and more. Apparently, the scientists and geneticists at TNI discovered people with Down syndrome don't necessarily metabolize foods and vitamins the way other people do. They have different needs, so they developed a nutritional supplement present in ratios appropriate for Down syndrome metabolism to help do what their bodies don't always do on their own. I read story after story about how well these children, who were taking these supplements, were doing. These children were amazing! Some were learning at age level, others weren't, but all were living happy, healthier lives than many people previously thought possible. And all because of a specially formulated nutritional supplement! It wasn't a drug, and that was the most appealing part for me. I read everything I could on the subject, then called and got even more information. I was put through to the president of the company (which blew me away) and he spent almost an hour talking to me. He explained how these vitamins helped Down kids, and why they were so important. I was amazed that the president, of any company, would take time out of his busy schedule to talk to me, but even more amazed that these supplements were helping so many children.

And this is how my pilgrimage began. Armed with new hope and better information, Bill and I decided we would keep our baby, no matter what. All of this took place before we got the amnio results. We went from complete fear and ignorance to an open mind and new resolve. If this is what God had in store for us, then we would handle it. Yes, we *could* handle it. My friend Denise told me that with or without Down syndrome, our baby girl would be perfect. She pointed out, according to the Bible, that we are *all* created in the image of God, therefore, a child with Down syndrome would conform to His image just as much as the rest of us. Our baby would be perfectly created in whatever image God wanted her. In His image. This thought gave me great peace. Thanks, Denise.

Okay. I was ready for anything. We were ready for anything. Actually, Bill was miles ahead of me. Without reading or influence through detailed information, he wanted to keep this baby, no matter how bad or how bleak. He didn't care. He loved this little girl, no matter what.

When my doctor called that Friday night, we didn't cry. We didn't cringe. I knew, somehow I just knew, that the tests had come back positive that our little girl did, in fact, have Down syndrome, and it was okay. *I was okay. Bill was okay.* We didn't panic. We called our family and friends, and it turned out that *we* were the ones comforting *them.* In two short days we had completely changed our way of thinking. We would do this, and we would do it well.

CHAPTER 2:

THE NEXT STEP

First thing I did on Monday morning was to call back the people at International Nutrition (TNI). I asked if there was anything I could do, now, while I was pregnant to help my baby. I learned they had recently developed a pre-natal supplement that could help my daughter's development in-utero. They sent me a list of the ingredients, which I showed to my doctor. She sent it to a colleague of hers who is a geneticist. His response was incredibly positive, which I must admit, actually surprised me. It's been my understanding, that the nutritional community and the medical community don't always see eye to eye. He assured us that because it was a nutritional supplement and not a drug, it wouldn't cause any harm to my unborn baby. So in a worse case scenario, even if it didn't help her, it wouldn't hurt her. So, within a week, I was taking the Nutrivene pre-natal vitamin, along with an iron supplement prescribed by my doctor. Her only regret was that there wasn't more information available for pregnant women carrying Down babies. She told me statistics showed that over 90% of women who found out that the baby they were carrying had Down syndrome, terminated their pregnancies. I couldn't believe it! But most people, when they hear the words Down syndrome, run away in fear. I refused to be one of them. And these statistics are not reserved only for Down Syndrome, but most any disability that is diagnosed in-utero results in termination.

The fifth and sixth months of my pregnancy were mostly uneventful. I continued to have regular check-ups with my doctor, but now I saw Dr. King as well. I was monitored closely by both, and my pregnancy continued to progress normally. It was decided that I would also meet with another OBGYN in Portland, as I would need to deliver my baby there. Our local hospital was not equipped to handle a high risk delivery like mine, so additional plans were being put into place.

Aside from appointments, I spent much of my time learning everything I could about Down syndrome. I read as many books as time allowed. I spoke to many mothers of Down children, and was so encouraged by most of their stories. My favorite phone call was to Cindy Wesner, a mother of a five year old boy named Joshua. She told me how her young child had touched so many peoples' lives. How his positive outlook had helped her become a better person. And then, she said something I'll never forget. She said that if Jesus were to come to her house today and offer to cure Joshua, like He did back in Biblical times, she would ask Him to fix his heart. He had had numerous heart surgeries and heart problems, and she would welcome Jesus to that. But she said she would never even consider asking Jesus to "fix" his Down syndrome, as that was just a part of who he was. She didn't consider the Down syndrome something that needed to be fixed.

Compare this to the story of another woman I called. When I spoke with this woman, the first thing I asked her was if she could tell me which books she had found most helpful and useful. She told me she had never read a book on Down syndrome. She went on to tell me, her five year old daughter with Down syndrome was both mentally and physically behind her 'normal' two year old. I've come to hate the word 'normal' but I'll get to that later. She wasn't potty trained, couldn't speak, and she could sit up but not walk. She told me, "That's just the way it is with Down kids.", and went on to say that I shouldn't expect too much from my own daughter. She also told me that she didn't belong to any support groups, because they were just a waste of time.

I couldn't get off the phone fast enough! The woman had never read a book about Down syndrome!! Instead she chose to live with her own pre-conceived notions, and her daughter was, thus, being punished because of her mothers' ignorance. She had no expectations for her daughter, was doing nothing to help her daughter, so she was left to fend for herself. This way of thinking is inconceivable to me!

How many children would learn to read and write if no one taught them how? How many children would learn to speak if no one spoke to them?

My oldest daughter Jackie, who was 11 at the time, wore glasses. We discovered she was having trouble seeing when she was 4, so we took her to an optometrist. The optometrist found her to have a vision problem, and fitted her with glasses. Could you imagine how different her life would be today had we let her fend for herself?

Had we said "Oh well, she can't see well so we won't expect too much." She wouldn't have done well in school because she wouldn't have been able to see the words in her books clearly, or the writing on the blackboard. She wouldn't be able to play sports well because athleticism requires coordination, which in turn requires good eyesight. But we chose instead to help her see better, which to us was a "no-brainer" decision.

The same way of thinking applied to my unborn child. I spoke to many doctors, nurses, and parents before she was born. I found out that the state of Oregon would provide her with *free* services, known as Early Intervention. She was eligible for a nurse to come to our house weekly to monitor her weight and health. She could also receive Physical Therapy from another specialist who would come to our house on a bi-weekly basis. Speech and Occupational therapy would also be available as she got older. By making these phone calls and doing this research, I was able to have all of this in place before my baby was even born.

I also spent time talking to my friends, telling them the news. Some people cried, or told me how sorry they were. Most expressed their sympathies, as if there had already been a death. Very few people said anything remotely comforting, except my closest friends. I remember the day I told my friend Margo, in a parking lot of all places. She hugged me and told me it would be okay, and that *we* could handle this. My friends Debbie and Denise said many a prayer for me, and were always just a phone call away if I needed them. Bill's parents were incredibly supportive. His mother cried when we first told her, but stood strong throughout my pregnancy. Actually,

Bill's parents were amazing. Bill describes his mother as "always rooting for the underdog". There was never any doubt in her mind about bringing this baby into the world. Like a lion protecting her cub, she puffed out her chest and stood tall, commenting that she would love this child with all her heart. Not in spite of her differences, but because of them. Bill's father was a beacon of strength and support, always ready to help in any way. Even *my* mother came around. She let go of some of her fears and became incredibly supportive of my pregnancy. Although, still not sure what to expect, or what the future would bring, she was there for me 100%.

Now all that was left to do was wait for the birth. Unfortunately, we didn't get to wait long enough.

CHAPTER 3:

READY OR NOT

It was a Sunday evening in September, and I felt terrible. I figured it was the seventh month blues, and I went upstairs to lie down. A friend of mine stopped by, and I didn't even come down to say hi. By Monday morning I was feeling bad enough to call my doctor. The receptionist informed me that she didn't have any appointments available, and I informed her that I was coming in anyway.

Bill took the day off of work, and drove me to the doctor's office. I'm sure I complained the entire way, as the pain in my abdomen seemed to be worsening by the minute. After waiting for what seemed like an eternity, actually 45 minutes, I told the receptionist that I needed to see the doctor, NOW! I made a big enough scene that she took me back to an examining room, where I informed the nurse that I couldn't wait any longer. Something, I knew, was terribly wrong. The nurse rushed out, and minutes later my doctor showed up. I remember lying back so she could push on my belly. I remember the look on her face when she told me I was in labor. I remember thinking she must be wrong, as I wasn't due for two more months. She immediately sent me to the local hospital, in hopes of stabilizing me and keeping me pregnant.

The first thing they did there was an ultrasound. The ultrasound showed that the baby had fluid trapped under her skin. She was inflating, almost like a balloon, from all of the fluid. This condition is called hydrops. Going into labor was nature's way of telling me, that my baby needed help. Fortunately, no one told me that hydrops was often fatal.

Next I was put into a bed with an IV in my arm and monitors strapped around my belly. I was quickly given a shot of terbutaline. This was supposed to quiet down pre-term labor, while making the patient feel high on caffeine. Then I was given a steroid shot, which would help the baby's lungs develop more fully incase the labor couldn't be stopped. The steroids needed at least 48 hours to do their job, so keeping me pregnant *at least* that long was crucial.

While the terbutaline did make me feel quite jittery, it didn't stop my labor. Next thing I knew, I was being sent by ambulance to Doernbecher Children's Hospital, Oregon Health and Sciences University. This is a large hospital, located two hours away in Portland. As I mentioned before, the hospital in the small town we lived in was not equipped to handle my type of high risk pregnancy. The cardiologist and other specialists I'd been seeing would all be waiting for me there. It was the bumpiest, most awful ride of my life.

There I was in pre-term labor, lying on my back on a cot, which was strapped to the floor of the ambulance/van. There were EMT's with me, monitoring whatever it is that they monitor. All the while we're speeding through town, around traffic, over bumps and around turns, with the siren blaring in my ears. Not fun.

About 3 hours later I was settled into yet another hospital bed, and I was given a magnesium drip to help calm my labor. It's a heavy dosage of metal, which does quiet down labor, but with staggering side effects. I was dizzy, nauseous, and vomiting. –I'm sure that's a visual you could have done without.– I couldn't walk or even sit up without help. The magnesium made my mouth so dry it was painful, and I wasn't allowed any water or fluids, only ice chips. I remember begging my husband to smuggle me in some water, which he did a couple of times, until we got caught. The charge nurse made me a deal: every time I peed, he'd give me a little water. In order to pee someone had to actually lift me out of bed and onto a portable potty they had wheeled into the center of my room.– Another special little visual.– So much for privacy, or dignity.

The magnesium did manage to keep me pregnant, but my contractions never stopped. I was in constant pain. In the midst of all this, I was given daily ultrasounds to check on the baby, and frequent echo-cardiograms to check on her heart. I was surrounded by doctors, cardiologists, perinatalogists, my new OBGYN, and specialists from every corner of the hospital.

Five more days passed, with more specialists, more exams, more tests, and always, more magnesium. I was miserable, but determined. The pain in my lower back was excruciating, and I drifted in and out of sleep. Jackie came and stayed with me for the weekend, so Bill could go home to take care of things. Jessi, who was 3 years old at the time, was staying with Bill's parents and luckily didn't have to see me like this. Justin, who was 13, was staying with family friends.

Jackie spent the weekend just hanging out with me, watching movies and rubbing my lower back. She is truly a gift, a really amazing kid. The drugs they were giving me to ease my pain didn't seem to help, but the pressure from a back rub provided some relief.

When Bill came back at the end of the weekend to pick up Jackie, and take over back-rubbing chores, the doctors told him they were going to keep me indefinitely, at least three more weeks. I begged him to go home, to take care of our children and to go back to work. Grudgingly and after much persuasion, he went.

Then I was truly alone. This wasn't a bad thing, as it gave me time to reflect. A lot had happened in the last few months of my life, none of which I had asked for or expected. Bill and I had not been trying to get pregnant, and although we were thrilled, we were still rebounding from all of the medical issues that had been thrown at us.

I thought back to when I first found out that my baby would not be 'normal' and how much I've come to hate that word. Who decides what is and isn't normal? Why is it that so many people, including doctors, use that word to describe a child that is not disabled? What gives anyone the right to say, that just because a child is different, they aren't normal? I laid there wondering how I was going to handle all of the chaos that was on its way into my life. I'd never faced anything this monumental before, and I was supposed to have two more months to prepare myself. More time to read, to learn, and to understand. More time for my fetus to grow and develop, to increase her chances for survival. More time.

It was then that Dr. Carey Winkler, my new Portland based OBGYN, came into my room. He'd been down the hall with another patient, and came by just to check on me (he'd already examined me twice). He asked me if I really wanted this baby, putting extra emphasis on the words 'really wanted'. I assured him, I did. I wasn't going through all of the motions just to please someone else, or because I was afraid of what people might think if I didn't.

He shared with me then how unfair he felt life could be some times. He told me about a patient down the hall, without using her name, of course. He told me of how she had armed guards outside of her room because she was on temporary leave from jail. She didn't care one bit about the baby she was about to deliver. Then he told me about another patient who was a few years older than me, who was about to lose the baby that she and her husband had spent years trying to conceive. We talked about why things happened, and why a woman from jail could have a healthy baby, and this other woman could not. We didn't find answers to these questions, but it helped both of us to try. And he gave me his word that he would do everything in his power to help me and my baby, and I believed him.

The next morning I was taken downstairs for yet another ultrasound. The transport attendant left me laying there in the hall outside the ultrasound room, as if I were some sort of package being delivered. When Dr. Winkler walked by, he couldn't believe it. There I was in the hall, crying and in pain. Still, the pain. It wouldn't go away. No one seemed to care that I was just waiting there, except Dr. Winkler. Immediately he got things moving, and all the specialists, my new best friends, were soon huddled around me and the buzzing ultrasound machine. The doctors discovered that the hydrops had worsened, and they needed to make a decision. They could go in with a long skinny needle right through my belly and insert it under the baby's skin and try to drain some of the fluid (that sounded fun). Or they could allow the baby to be born, and then try the same procedure with far fewer possible complications.

Because the hydrops was worsening quickly, they chose to allow me to give birth. That meant they could turn off the magnesium, which was the happiest moment since my arrival at the hospital 6 days ago. I called Bill, and after being home for less than 12 hours, he was on his way back. The children had to be shuffled off again to friends' houses. What a mess I was making of everyone's lives.

By the time Bill arrived, they had put me on pitocin, which is a drug that is given to quicken up labor. So they spent the first 6 days giving me drugs so I *wouldn't* give birth, and now they were giving me drugs *to* give birth. It was all so surreal. My cardiologist and my OBGYN (notice how I now *own* them!) checked on me constantly. After everyone was updated and 'in place' I was given the long awaited epidural, and finally, some relief. Actually, the first epidural didn't help, so I was given another. Lucky me.

Unfortunately, the birth didn't happen quickly. While we waited, one of the head doctors from the NICU (neo-natal intensive care unit) came in to give Bill and me a dose of reality. She explained that if our baby was born this early, her chances for survival would be slim. The combination of her heart defects and Down syndrome were severe enough on their own, but coupled with the hydrops and a premature birth...well, it was bleak at best.

That's when I tuned out. All I heard were the muffled sounds and BLAH, BLAH, BLAH, BLAH while she continued her speech. Bill listened intently and asked questions, and actually understood everything they discussed. Later, when she finally left the room, we decided not to let her little speech scare us. We knew she was speaking the truth, as she saw it, from her medical point of view. But we were absolutely certain this child would live, and that was that. We hadn't come this far to lose her now. We didn't need to discuss it further. We were calm. We were certain. I can't even explain this in any way that makes sense. We had been given an incredible peace about her birth, and we refused to let anyone, even a doctor of her merit, shake our faith.

Later, when the time was imminent, an intern arrived and stood in my room, armed with a warm blanket. His job was to whisk the newborn baby away into the NICU, where all the specialists would be waiting, and where she would be pricked, probed, checked, tested, and hopefully, kept alive.

Jenessa Dominique Sherman was born at 8:35 am on September

14, 1999. She was taken from me so quickly that I didn't even get to see her, let alone hold her. I sent Bill with her to watch and observe, but mostly just to be there with her. I had to be cleaned up, sewn up, and all those other lovely little things that happen after giving birth. And I needed that time to just lay there. To be out of pain and just to *lay there,* and absorb everything that had happened in the last week of my life.

CHAPTER 4:

BABY J

Within minutes of being whisked into the NICU, Jenessa had needles thrust into both sides of her body. They were sucking out the excess fluid from her chest, to make enough room for her lungs to be able to expand, inflate, and breathe. Without this procedure she would have died – immediately, as she would have been unable to take a breath. She was intubated (breathing with the help of a ventilator) had IV's attached to the blood vessels in her umbilical cord, had a feeding tube (called a nasogastric,or NG-tube) inserted, had an echocardiogram, and more. By the time I was wheeled in to see her a couple of hours after her birth, I could hardly find her underneath all of those tubes and wires. I remember looking up at Bill and whispering,"She's so cute. I didn't expect her to be so cute". She was quite puffy from all the extra fluid, but managed to be cute in spite of it.

When first weighed, born 8 weeks early, Jenessa weighed 5 lbs. 15 oz. After they drained all the fluid from her, she weighed only 4 lb. 8 oz. I couldn't even imagine that she could still look so puffy after losing so much fluid, but she did.

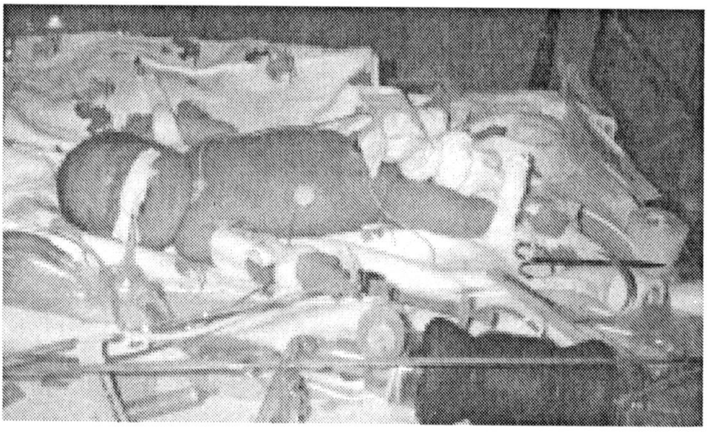

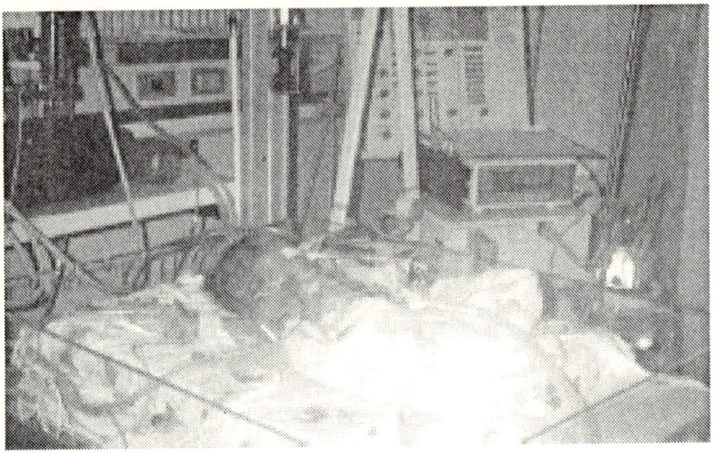

Jenessa at birth, somewhere under all those wire

Jenessa was in an incubator next to another child, of the same gestational age. That child weighed less than 2 pounds, and was the tiniest baby I'd ever seen. Jenessa was so much bigger, and looked so much healthier, even with her heart condition and the Down syndrome. I had to wonder, could it be the Nutrivene? Could I, taking those special pre-natal vitamins, have helped Jenessa be so strong, in spite of everything? Was God watching over my little girl, listening to our prayers? I believe, yes, on both counts, and not necessarily in that order.

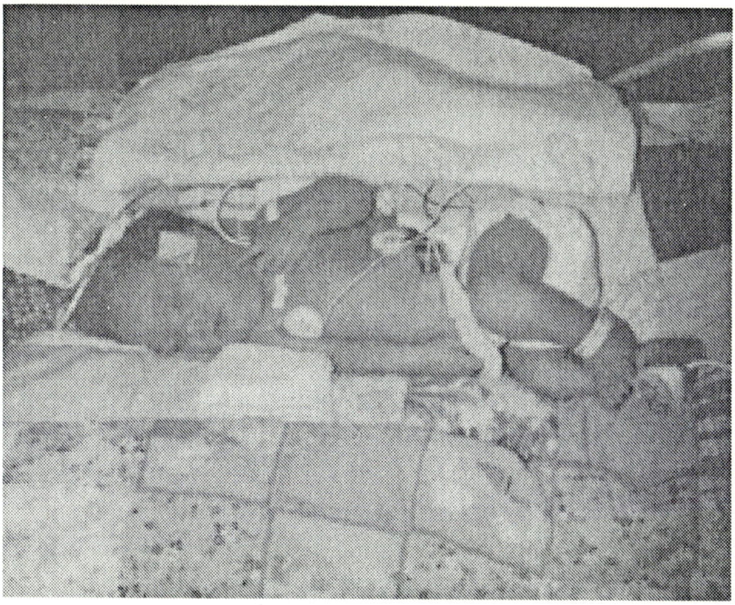

Jenessa at 4 days old, after all the fluid had been drained.

Georgia Ditzenberger was the NICU Nurse Practitioner who was in charge of Jenessa's care. Below is what she wrote about those first days, and then weeks, of Jenessa's life.

> Jenessa was born to a 39 year old, gravida 4, para 2, now 3, mother with an in utero diagnosis of Trisomy 21, hydrops, AVC, and TOF. This is the beginning of the discharge dictation in which I summarized Jenessa's hospitalization on the day she went home, October 11, 1999. The summary is clinically oriented and full of medical jargon that effectively encapsulates Jenessa's stay with us in the DNCC but it doesn't capture the true human reality of the situation.
>
> By the time I met Jenessa and her family on

September 27, 1999, she had been in the DNCC since her birth on September 14. She had gone through resuscitation after birth, requiring bag-mask ventilation and then very soon after birth, intubation (insertion of an endotracheal, or breathing, tube into her trachea through her mouth) to help her to breathe effectively. Two catheters were inserted into her freshly cut umbilical cord, one into the vein and the other into an artery, to allow pain-free blood draws and a stable access for intravenous fluids and, later, parenternal nutrition. Jenessa had bilateral pleural effusions or fluid surrounding her lungs within the pleural cavity, which needed to be removed by inserting a needle on either side of her chest; 30cc of excess fluid was removed from her right chest and 90cc from her left chest. Fluid reaccummulated around her left lung, which necessitated another procedure to remove it and a chest tube placed to allow for continuous drainage to occur until it finally subsided on September 20. The chest tube remained in, however, as Jenessa then developed a pneumothorax (air outside the lung, essentially in the same area as the fluid had been) which was alleviated by evacuation via the chest tube. Her pneumothorax resolved within the next day or so and the chest tube was finally removed on the 21st. Throughout this time, Jenessa had been requiring the assistance of a ventilator, which was providing her support and additional breaths via her endotracheal tube. The endotracheal tube was removed September 19 when she was breathing effectively enough on her own.

Jenessa's heart condition was assessed and monitored by our pediatric cardiologists. She was diagnosed as having Tetralogy of Fallot variant—

AV Canal with pulmonic stenosis and an overriding aorta. She had five echocardiograms during her first hospital stay. The cardiologists recommended that her oxygen saturations should remain within the 80s, but no less than 75, to maintain her cardiac status until her first surgical intervention. Initially following the removal of the endotracheal tube, Jenessa maintained saturations in the 80's on room air but developed an oxygen requirement the day I met her, September 27. When she was discharged home on October 11, she required 150cc, or just over 1/8 lpm of oxygen through her nasal cannula to maintain her saturations in the 80s. The goal of such monitoring and oxygen therapy was to provide time for Jenessa to grow large enough to improve her tolerance of the necessary surgeries.

Nutrition was a vital part of Jenessa's treatment. Babies with heart conditions require increased calories to adequately grow and often tire quickly when eating. Jenessa was also born at 32 weeks gestation, or 8 weeks premature, and weighed 2705 grams. She was hydropic at birth, a condition in which there was excess fluid in both her tissues and, as previously discussed, in her pleural cavities. We had to estimate her "dry" weight of about 2000 grams, based on her general length, size, and weight averages for other infants of her gestational age at birth. We used this weight to calculate her fluid and caloric intake while she lost the excess fluid and also while she began to take on real weight gains with enhanced caloric intake. Once she passed this weight, we used her daily weight to make appropriate adjustments. By the time we became acquainted, Jenessa was nippling what she could and then being fed the rest by a continuous infusion through a small and very pliable gavage tube that went through her nose down into her stomach. She needed to have enhanced calorie food: formula with added hydrolyzed fat to increase the calories from the typical newborn formula of 20 calories/ounce to 26 calories/ounce. She began gaining weight of about 15 – 30 grams (~1/2 – 1 ounce) per day on this regimen.

Jenessa was placed on the NNP (Neo-natal nurse practitioner) service when we began our 2 month on-service time on September 27th. Every morning either the other NNP, Susan, or myself would come to Jenessa's bedside and give her a physical; she would squirm and wiggle while we listened to her heart and breath sounds, and gently press on her stomach, then check her pulses and reflexes. She was very responsive and would listen to me talk to her for brief moments during her physical. Her parents, Debbie and Bill, were very involved in her care; Debbie spent hours daily at the hospital, even though it meant a 4 hour round trip each visit, while Bill worked at their restaurant on the coast and took care of their older children, coming when he could to visit also. We talked daily about Jenessa's medical plan of care, as well as her future needs and surgeries. By the time Jenessa was ready to leave for home, she was on a plan of care that would promote optimal growth while she waited for her first surgery and her parents were prepared to take on the responsibility of her care.

Working with Debbie while we formulated Jenessa's home care was a very interesting and rewarding experience. She was very willing to ask questions and listened to the answers, never stopping until she understood as completely as possible the information given. She also would read and research topics on her own and would discuss what she had learned. She had researched Trisomy 21 while she was pregnant and had prepared herself as much as she could for what life may hold for herself and her family when the new baby arrived. She researched mega-vitamin therapy for infants with Trisomy 21 and willingly brought in the information for us (the medical team) to peruse.

Jenessa was discharged home on October 11 with oxygen, respiratory-cardiac monitor and the feeding regimen as described above. She weighed 2545 grams. Initially she did well and gained weight. She returned to the DNCC and the NNP service on October 18 for de-compensation in which she became apneic (stopped breathing), lethargic, and required stimulation to restart breathing. Her parents rushed her to the local hospital and she was emergently transported by a specialized pediatric team to DNCC. During this hospitalization, after she was stabilized, the pediatric cardiologist decided to wait no longer for the first surgery and Jenessa was transferred to another hospital for that surgery on October 24.

Our friendship initially was limited by our professional relationship of NNP- patient's-parent while in the hospital but has grown personal since Jenessa was discharged from our unit.

Georgia R. Ditzenberger, MN, RNC, NNP
Doernbecher Neonatal Care Center
OHSU/Doernbecher Children's Hospitals

****

The day prior to Jenessa being discharged, we were asked to take an infant CPR class given there at the hospital. (Actually, they wouldn't let us take Jenessa home *unless* we had completed the course.) Bill, myself, and Justin took the course, while Jackie babysat Jessi in a nearby room. To me, it was terribly frightening. I didn't think I could do it! The nurses told me the standing joke was: If you take the course, odds were you'd never need it. I liked those odds. We also took a two hour training course on the heart/breathing monitor they would be sending Jenessa home on. This was even scarier than the CPR course. I'm not good with machines, and the thought of a machine being attached to my daughter at home didn't sit well with me. I wanted her to stay in the hospital until she no longer needed tubes, nurses, and machines. I wanted to be her mother, not her nurse.

Unfortunately, I was going to be *both.*

CHAPTER 5:

THE HOMECOMING

After what seemed like forever in the hospital, Jenessa was finally coming home. We sent out her birth announcement, along with a letter telling our friends about our special baby.

Jenessa was to be sent home with her NG-tube still in. This NG-tube, a nasogastric tube, is a clear plastic tube that is inserted through the nose, down the back of the throat, through the esophagus and ending in the stomach. I had been trained on how to remove it and clean it and re-insert it. *Much more than I ever wanted to learn.*

She would be sent home with various medications, which had to be carefully measured, and then given. She was still on oxygen, so I had to learn about that as well. She actually had an oxygen backpack that was to go with her everywhere, and then an actual tank had been brought to our house. But the worst part, the very worst part, was that she would need to be on a special heart monitor at night. This measures, counts, and waits for each breath. It would alarm us if she were to stop breathing. Even though Bill and I had gone through the special training for this, I was still completely against having it. It scared me to death. I didn't want it, but the nurses convinced me that it would be better to be safe, than sorry. We also came home with a special feeding pump, which, when hooked up to Jenessa's NG-tube, would actually pump formula into her at a very slow pace overnight. She wasn't strong enough yet to eat normally, as she still couldn't suck down more than 5 cc's at a time. (5 cc's is equal to 1 teaspoon, and obviously, that wouldn't be enough to sustain her.) By hooking Jenessa up to this special feeding pump, she would be fed very small amounts at a time, distributed at even intervals throughout the night (It operates on the same principle as an IV). During the day, when it was time to eat, I could bottle feed her as much as she could take, and then feed her the rest through her NG-tube.

The most important part of feeding Jenessa was to make sure to keep what little food she actually ate, down. In other words, the object was to keep her from throwing up.

All of this terrified me. I had brought two other children home from the hospital, with my biggest worry being when/if they would sleep through the night. With Jenessa, my biggest worry was whether or not I'd be able to keep her alive. And I don't say this lightly, as it was exactly how I felt at the time.

"It's exactly how it was!"

Could we keep this fragile, beautiful little girl alive? Could we *grow* her big enough to have her open heart surgery that she so desperately needed to live? The doctors told us they hoped to do this surgery at about one year of age. But in order to do that with the utmost hope of success, she needed to weigh about 15 pounds. And she was coming home now weighing only 5 1/2 pounds. With a heart monitor. With oxygen. With a feeding tube. *With me.*

Jenessa was discharged on the 27th day of her life. My friend Debbie came to get us from the hospital. Debbie is an RN, so I felt a bit less nervous about the two hour drive home. We buckled Jenessa and me into the back seat, and Debbie drove. When we arrived at home, Debbie came in and helped me get the feeding pump ready for later. We got Jenessa snuggled nicely into her crib, and watched her sleep. Debbie stayed with me until I felt I could manage on my own, and then I just sat there and watched my baby girl. I watched her chest, to make certain she was breathing. I changed her diaper, which was no easy task with all the tubes everywhere. I was so nervous that I might pull a tube out, or dislodge something. Imagine, a mother of four, afraid to change her baby's diaper.

Bill came home a couple of hours later, and we managed to make it through the first day. The first night would be something far different.

First, I got the overnight formula bag ready--*that was the easy part*. Bill hooked up the heart monitor, as I was still too afraid of it. We held her, loved her, rocked her, and finally, put her to bed. I hooked up the feeding pump, and watched this machine start to feed my daughter. Again, a surreal feeling filled the room. This was out of some medical textbook, it shouldn't be happening in our home. But it was.

Jenessa slept through that first night at home. And the next, and the next one after that. I become more comfortable with all of her tubes. I could give her medication to her without reading the labels, as I'd memorized the amounts, and how to give them. When we were home, it was easier for Jenessa to just stay in her room, not to be moved too far from her crib. This way, I didn't have to unhook the oxygen tank and hook up the oxygen backpack; I could just leave her "attached". Every time anyone held her there had to be great care taken not to dislodge any of the tubes or wires. After all, if something came out or un-hooked, I would have to re-hook or re-attach something. This was way too scary of a thought.

Four days after Jenessa came home, I finally ventured out to the grocery store with the oxygen backpack intact. Somehow, with Bill's help, I was doing this.

But on the sixth day, something was wrong. Jenessa developed a fever, and was extremely fussy and uncomfortable. She threw up everything she ate. I gave her a cool bath, I gave her some Tylenol, I rocked her, but still, she was not alright. Of course, it was a Sunday, and all the doctors' offices were closed. Bill was at work. Jackie called him and insisted that he come home immediately.

While we were waiting for Bill to get home, Jenessa stopped breathing. I shook her, I screamed at her, and she took another breath.

By this time Bill was running up the stairs. Jackie was screaming at him to help, when Jenessa stopped breathing again. Bill gave her two rescue breaths, and she started to breathe. We called our local hospital, and this idiot of a doctor told us he thought we should drive her to Portland. Can you imagine, driving two hours through the mountains with a baby that might stop breathing again? We took her instead to the Emergency Room at the local hospital (we made sure to avoid that idiot doctor!) While trying to stabilize her, Jenessa went in and out of consciousness more times than I could count. Bill and I would be watching her heart rate on the monitors, and it would just drop. It would be at 150 bpm, then 140, 130, 120, go all the way down to 40, and 30. She was just lying there, dying. We would scream at her, shake her, and just yell until the bleeps on the screen started to go back up. She was dying before our eyes, and would have died right there on the table if it had not been for our constant efforts of yelling and shaking her. It was like we were *reminding* her to breathe, and *reminding* her to live. This went on for about an hour. She'd be doing okay, and then close her eyes like she was going to sleep, and her heart rate would drop again. It was a nightmare, except that it wasn't. This was real, and it was happening to our baby.

While everyone continued to work at stabilizing her, the head of the ER called the Panda Team from OHSU. The Panda Team is a group of doctors and nurses who specialize in treating infants. They came and picked up Jenessa and me in a specially equipped ambulance, and transported us back to the hospital which we had left just six short days before. During the drive, Jenessa continued to float in and out of consciousness. The doctors hovered over her, giving her oxygen and watching her every movement (or lack thereof). They did whatever it took on that scary drive to keep our daughter alive. We will be indebted to them forever, and we thank God every night for their competency.

Upon arrival, Jenessa was whisked back into the NICU, and I watched as the doctors and nurses went about their work.

When she was finally and completely stabile, I fell asleep in the waiting room next door.

The next morning, Georgia came to find me, and we just stood there and hugged. We didn't speak any words, as they didn't seem to be necessary. We went to Jenessa's room, and we both just stood there, and cried. She wasn't supposed to be back here. Not yet.

CHAPTER 6:

THE SHUNT

The specialists were assembled in no time. They determined that she would need heart surgery in order to survive. Jenessa needed a shunt (a modified Blalock-Taussig shunt, in case you really want to know) inserted into her heart, which would re-route blood to where it was supposed to be going on its own. They couldn't do the surgery until Jenessa was stronger. It was decided that she would stay and be monitored again in the NICU. She was out of danger, but still needed time to regain her strength.

Here, in Dr. King's own words, is why she needed the surgery, and what it would accomplish:

> Over the first weeks of life, Jenessa's echocardiograms revealed increasing right ventricular outflow tract obstruction. As a result, Jenessa's oxygen saturations continued to decline over the first several weeks of her life. Initially, this drop in saturation was attributed in part to Jenessa's fluid around her lungs, (i.e. her hydrops). However, as the hydrops improved her oxygen saturations (SAT's) continued to decline. In light of the decreasing oxygen saturations we were faced with the decision of either proceeding with a complete repair of her defect, which at only six pounds would carry an operative mortality of 15-20%. The other surgical option would be to proceed with a systemic to pulmonary artery shunt, which would temporarily improve Jenessa's blood flow. After discussion with her parents, we decided to proceed with the lower risk operation.

Six days later, with Jenessa at her strongest point yet, we were transferred to Legacy Emanuel Children's Hospital, which was only a few miles away. And the next day, Jenessa had her first open heart surgery. The shunt was implanted, and the surgery was a success. Four hours later, Jenessa was wheeled into the PICU, (pediatric intensive care unit). This would become our new home.

We could hardly see our daughter, as there were tubes everywhere. Nurses and doctors and specialists once again took center stage in our lives.

Jenessa did so well that the doctors decided to extubate her (remove her breathing tube) the very next day. Unfortunately, she stopped breathing and had to be reintubated. No one had been expecting this, and I was sent out of the room while doctors and nurses scrambled to keep her alive. We had to wait six long days before they tried again to extubate her, and this time was without incident.

Dr. King explains this first surgery:

> Jenessa's surgery consisted of incising the sternum (i.e. the breast bone) which then permitted exposure of the outside of the heart and great vessels which exited the heart. In Jenessa's case, the plan was to place a small tube of gortex (referred to as a shunt) between the aorta and the pulmonary artery. This procedure would increase blood flow to the lungs and then allow Jenessa's oxygen saturations to increase to a safe level, so that she could grow and develop. During the operation the innominate artery, which is the first branch off the aorta, was isolated and a clamp was placed on the vessel. A 3.5 mm piece of gortex was then sewn into the artery. The right pulmonary artery was isolated and the clamp was placed over a portion of the right pulmonary and the other end of the tube was sewn in place.

> Once the two ends of the shunt were sewn into place the clamps were removed and the shunt was opened. Following this operation, Jenessa's saturations increased from 75% to 90%.
>
> Following the operation her saturations did increase as expected. However, she did develop some pulmonary congestion which is common with children who undergo palliative surgery rather than corrective surgeries. When the arteries to the lung receive insufficient blood flow they are smaller than normal. When the blood flow is suddenly increased to the lungs, infants frequently develop pulmonary congestion for the first few days after a shunt procedure. In Jenessa's case she did develop this pulmonary congestion and required assistance on the ventilator for approximately six days. After she was taken off of the ventilator the congestion in her lungs stabilized with a combination of digoxin and diuretics. Our long term plan then was to help Jenessa grow and develop until the time in which we could proceed with her corrective surgery.

Then, a week later, Jenessa came home. Again. The good news was, she no longer needed to be hooked up to the heart monitor, and she no longer required oxygen. This meant she could actually leave her bedroom without having to drag around an oxygen tank/backpack. The only clue (to an outsider) that she wasn't quite well was her NG-tube, which would be a part of her pretty little face for many months to come. Thank goodness for my friend Debbie, the nurse. She came over every week to move the tube from one side of her nose to the other. I'd been trained on how to do it, but I just couldn't bear to cause my baby so much pain. It was awful; not only did she scream, but she would arch her back in pain. Debbie wasn't thrilled to be doing this either, but she was medically trained to do it, and was happy to be able to help. This worked great until the time Jenessa pulled it out herself and Debbie was nowhere to be found. Imagine, she actually had a life other than helping me with my own child. But I surprised myself by getting it 'in' on my first try. I had become more of a nurse than I gave myself credit for.

Now I could rest easier. The surgery was a 'temporary fix'. It would keep her breathing and her blood moving where the doctors wanted it to go-*this is helpful!*. This homecoming was much less eventful than the first one, for which I was grateful.

My days became fairly normal. I bottle fed Jenessa with the smallest bottle you've ever seen, and supplemented additional formula through her NG-tube. I started her on the Nutrivene supplements, as she was not able to be on them while hospitalized. It was so nice to have a baby that wasn't hooked up to an oxygen tank; we could go to the store and run our errands with minimal effort these days! At night, I did have to hook Jenessa up to the feeding pump, which I mastered in no time. Because it fed her continuously throughout the night, she slept through the night from the start. Her heart still didn't work normally, so she tired quicker than a baby without any heart problems. A good night's sleep was essential....for all of us.

Weeks turned into months, and Jenessa did fabulous. She grew, albeit slowly, and she quickly became aware of her surroundings and her family. When she was two months old, the two pastors from our church came to visit. As they were leaving, Jenessa looked at me and smiled. Tears ran down my face. My daughter, who wasn't supposed to live, *knew* me! I realized on that very day how much I loved this little girl. I think it took me so long because I had been protecting myself. I had been so afraid of losing her, then so concentrated on caring for her special needs. Now, it seemed, I could relax and just love her.

We had weekly home visits from Lynn, our local county health nurse. Lynn and I became fast friends, and we played little games where we'd guess Jenessa's weight each week. It was hard for her to gain weight, as she spent more calories and more energy than normal because of her heart defects. Sucking her bottle actually cost her more calories than she got from the formula, so it was an uphill battle for her to gain even an ounce. This was compounded by what we thought was reflux disease. Jenessa threw up *all the time.* Because of all of her health issues, it didn't dawn on us until Jenessa was about 2 months old that maybe she was allergic to the milk. When you have a sick child, your brain doesn't seem to go to the easy, normal fixes. I had read so many books about Down syndrome, and every book listed reflux as a possible characteristic, so I just assumed that explained it. But when Bill reminded me that all three of our other children had had milk allergies as infants– *duh*!. I flew out of the house, drove like a crazy woman to the grocery store, and bought a container of soy formula. She stopped throwing up that very night, and slowly started to gain weight.

We also had visits, bi-monthly, from Mary Ann, who is the Physical Therapist for our county. She moved around Jenessa's little arms and legs, and helped her with strength and movement. Then came Vera, an Occupational Therapist, who helped with her fine motor skills. Then came the Speech Therapist, who did absolutely nothing but inform me of all the things my daughter would never do. Needless to say, I soon had no respect for this woman.

All of these visits became a part of our normal routine. We had regular check-ups with a pediatrician as well, but this woman was clueless, and began to suggest unnecessary treatments and surgeries. She told me that the vitamin supplements I was giving Jenessa were a waste of time and offered me false hope where there was no hope to be had. I should have just faced the fact that my daughter has Down syndrome and will never be normal. I had already faced that fact! I wasn't giving her the vitamins in an effort to cure her; I didn't feel she needed to be cured. I was giving her the vitamins in an effort to keep her healthy, nothing more. I've devoted an entire chapter to this doctor and the speech therapist later in the book.

By December, we were pretty much a normal family again. We went to my in-laws for Christmas, where Jenessa seemed fussy and not herself. Her breathing appeared labored, but I wrote it off to grandparents, aunts, uncles, cousins,...you know, all the commotion that is involved with Christmas. We left early though because she just didn't seem quite right.

Two days later, I brought her car seat into the house, where I buckled her in safely, for an excursion to the grocery store. I know, my life is *way* too exciting. I was home alone with her, and we were going off to hit the after Christmas sales. I left her in her car seat on the living room floor, and went out to warm up the car. When I returned, about 30 seconds later, I picked up the car seat...AND JUST KNEW!...she wasn't breathing. I unbuckled her, shook her, yelled at her, pounded on her little back.....and nothing happened. She was starting to turn blue and her body was becoming rigid. I put her on the couch and started CPR. Again, nothing happened. I frantically called my husband at work and told him that Jenessa wasn't breathing, and I needed help. I hung up, and continued with the CPR. Bill called 911. I was yelling at her, yelling at God, and begging Him to let her live. Finally, after almost ten minutes, she started to make this horrendous sputtering sound. It sounded like air was coming out of her ears. It wasn't, but it wasn't coming out right. The noise got worse, and louder, and I didn't know if she was dying or coming back to life. I am certain, absolutely certain, that Jenessa had died during these ten minutes. Next thing I knew, she was breathing, badly. Loud gasping noises, loud noises that sounded like some sort of whistle. Noises meant Jenessa was back! Just then the EMT's ran into my living room, cut open her shirt, and took over. Bill was right behind them. They could see she was in bad shape; they put her on oxygen and did what they could to stabilize her. Then, they made the necessary phone calls, and put us both in an ambulance and whisked us to the local hospital.

Upon arrival, she was hooked up to all sorts of monitors. Her breathing still wasn't right, and they desperately wanted to give her this special drug through an IV. The problem was, no one could get an IV started. She was still so small, and no one there was trained in infant IV's. Every time they poked her to try and get the IV threaded, she would scream and kick, and she would get so angry she would stop breathing. After about the fourth time, I lost it. I screamed at everyone there in the ER, and told them they had to stop hurting my daughter. Obviously, they weren't smart enough to see the correlation between poking her with needles and then her breathing stopping. Her SAT's (oxygen saturations) were all over the place, and there was another nurse giving her too much oxygen. He insisted that he needed to keep her SAT's in the 90-100 range, (a healthy person without a heart defect usually SAT's around 100) and we insisted that the 70's were the right range for her. Then the head ER doctor contacted Dr. King in Portland, who quickly confirmed that her SAT's didn't need to be so high. Hmmmm....Imagine that, we, her parents were right? In the meantime, Lynn Archibald, the head pharmacist, entered the room. He had heard the call come in about a baby being brought in who wasn't breathing, and he figured it was us. His daughters, Brenna and Jenna, are best friends with my oldest daughter Jackie, so we knew Lynn well. He arrived in the midst of my screaming fit. He assured everybody there that he could put that drug, I don't know what it was, I just know that they insisted she needed it, immediately, into a shot. He ran out of the ER, and appeared back minutes later with the shot. Problem solved.

In talking with the head of the Emergency Room, Dr. King felt he probably didn't even need to see Jenessa, as it appeared that the local doctors had everything under control. He assumed it wasn't anything too serious, and told us not to worry too much. He thought maybe she had simply choked on something, and that was what had caused her to stop breathing.

During all of this, the radiologist brought Jenessa's x-rays into the ER. The doctors shuffled off into another room to look them over. Bill followed the doctors, even though they hadn't invited either of us to join them. Remember, we're the 'stupid parents'. While in the room, Bill was the one who noticed that Jenessa's heart was swollen to about twice her normal size. Bill insisted that they go get the x-rays from our last visit and he demanded comparison of the two x-rays be viewed by the doctors. Bill was the one who knew our baby's heart, and what it was supposed to look like.

This information changed everything. Upon hearing this, Dr. King immediately decided to send a Life flight helicopter to pick Jenessa up and transport her to Legacy Emanuel Children's Hospital, where he and the other specialists would be waiting. So while Bill waited for the Life flight crew, I went home and packed a bag. Bill came home as soon as Jenessa was safely put into the helicopter, and we drove to Portland in shock.

CHAPTER 7:

HERE WE GO AGAIN

Two hours later we were back in the PICU of Legacy Emanuel Children's Hospital. My favorite nurse, Jennie Peterson, had been assigned to Jenessa's room, which was an immediate relief. Dr. King was there; of course he was, where else would he be? It was as if he just magically appeared whenever we needed him, as if Jenessa was his only patient. He was giving her an echocardiogram, and he looked strained and more than a bit worried. I didn't always understand the 'cardiac stuff' he explained about her condition, but I had come to understand that when he was happy, I was happy. He did not look happy, *at all.*

He explained that a tremendous amount of damage had been done to her heart, because she had stopped breathing for so long. There was no way he could know if she had incurred any sort of brain damage, but that too was entirely possible. He went on to discuss the ejection fraction of her heart, which is defined like this:

> --The pumping efficiency of the heart is evaluated using a measurement called ejection fraction. The ejection fraction of the heart is the fraction or proportion of blood that the heart pumps (ejects) out of the left ventricular chamber with each heartbeat. People with a normal, healthy heart typically have an ejection fraction of about 50-55%. This means that 55% of the blood that fills the left ventricle is pumped out to the body with each contraction. The left ventricle never completely pumps out all the blood, just a fraction of it. A low ejection fraction is one of the key indicators used to identify people who are at risk for sudden cardiac arrest.

Dr. King told us that Jenessa's ejection fraction was now at 10%. Bluntly, he explained that if, over the next 48 hours, her heart's ejection fraction improved to even 11%, she would, probably, live. If it declined to even 9%, she would, most likely, die; at which point, her only hope for survival would be a heart transplant. He advised us that getting her a heart for transplant would be next to impossible, as her Down syndrome would preclude her from being chosen as a recipient.

I knew he didn't look happy when we arrived, but I had no idea it was this bad. This was the first time that Dr. King ever talked about my baby dying. We had asked for the truth, and we were speechless.

Bill asked what her chances were, and we were told that she had as much of a chance of making it through the night as not. That translated into a 50/50 chance. These were not the odds we were hoping for.

We watched as nurses and doctors and respiratory therapists worked on Jenessa, all playing their important roles in saving her life. She'd already been intubated, as this was the best chance her heart would have to rest and relax. If the machine could breathe for her, it would give her heart a chance to rest and possibly grow stronger. They wouldn't test her heart again for 48 hours, as there needed to be enough time allowed for there to be improvement, or, God forbid, for it to decline further. All that was left for Bill and I to do was wait. And pray.

We spent the night on cots in a special room set up for families of patients by the PICU. We took turns staying with Jenessa, and trying to get some sleep, but neither was very productive. Jenessa was resting comfortably, and all we could do was watch as the ventilator pumped air in and out of her lungs. Doctors checked on her periodically, as did nurses and the respiratory therapists who came in every few hours to beat on her chest. Actually, they used a special instrument to pound on her chest, in an effort to keep mucus from forming and clogging her airway.

By morning we were exhausted. Mostly from the shock of just

being in this predicament again. Yesterday, I was going shopping with my daughter, and today we didn't know if she was going to live.

After another meeting with Dr. King, we were convinced that she was stable and nothing else was going to happen today. I was able to persuade Bill to go home, again, try to muddle through work, and to be there for our other children. As always, I would stay….and wait.

I think this was my worst day since Jenessa had been born. There was nothing I could do, nothing the doctors could do, except wait. Her heart would either start to mend itself or it wouldn't. And we had to wait another day to do the test. It was the longest day of my life.

My friend Margo came to visit, mostly just to hold my hand. She had driven two hours over a mountain, in the midst of a wet Oregon winter, *was there any other kind?*, just to be with me. Words cannot express the gratitude I felt for her at this moment. Having a friend to talk to and just sit with on such a scary day was an incredible gift. Thanks, Margo.

After she left, I found myself alone again in Jenessa's room. I sat watching all the different monitors, which by now, I could read as well as any nurse. I was looking for any sign of improvement. I'm sure I did this for several hours, distracted only when a doctor or nurse entered the room. By the end of the day I was completely depressed. I couldn't eat, couldn't sleep, and my only form of entertainment came from the monotonous sounds made by the various machines keeping my baby alive.

I remember walking over to her crib, holding her tiny little hand, begging her to hang on. I prayed that God would help her, strengthen her heart, and let her live. I was looking down at her, watching her sleep, when she opened her eyes and smiled at me! Keep in mind she had a giant intubation tube down her throat, which was taped to her face. It was as if she was telling me not to worry, that everything was going to be 'okay'. And then she was asleep again, as if nothing miraculous had just happened. The doctors came and went, and day quietly turned to night. I managed to pull myself out of her room long enough to call Bill, to tell him not to worry. Somehow, Jenessa had managed to "tell" me she was going to be *al*right.

The next morning, Dr. King arrived early to do the test, to measure Jenessa's ejection fraction, again. Nurse Jennie assured me that if her heart measured anything over 10%, even one point, that would be considered a good sign. I was sent out of the room, to wait. You'd think with all this practice I'd be getting really good at it, but waiting, along with patience, has never been one of my strong suits.

It seemed like hours when I was finally called back into the room. First thing I did was look at Dr. King, trying to read his face, hoping for some hint of a good result, but, what I saw was confusion.

Jenessa's ejection fraction had measured at 24%! No one expected it to be so greatly improved. There were children who'd been hospitalized here for months, with their ejection fraction improving only 1% a week. It was taking them months to get where Jenessa had gotten in less than two days! I was overjoyed, relieved, excited, but not entirely surprised. Yesterdays smile had put me at ease, and today's results were nothing short of a miracle. My baby, my precious angel, was going to live! I silently thanked the Lord for not taking my little girl.

Two days later Dr. King tested her heart again. He told me not to expect as big of an improvement, so when the results came back at 48%, I actually saw him smile! If you knew this doctor, you'd understand the significance of this moment. This is the most dedicated, hardest working doctor I've ever known. He talks like a medical dictionary. He knows more about hearts, vessels, chambers, and blood than any medical textbook. He is brilliant beyond words. He was smiling!

Here, in Dr. King's own words, is what happened:

> Jenessa's "setback" came as a shock to all of us who were caring for her. I had seen Jenessa two weeks earlier and all appeared to be going well. Her oxygen saturations were stable at 84%,and her

weight gain was satisfactory as well. During the days prior to her respiratory arrest she had developed some recurrent vomiting, which in her case appeared to be related to esophageal reflux. (These are babies who have recurrent vomiting secondary to an incompetent valve between the stomach and the espophagus. Consequently, some babies regurgitate their food into their esophagus and this can ultimately affect their breathing.) In Jenessa's case she had been placed in her car seat just prior to her respiratory arrest. Jenessa likely stopped breathing because of some stomach contents which had regurgitated into her airway. Once she stopped breathing her heart rate slowed because of the lack of oxygen. As the heart rate slowed, Jenessa's blood pressure continued to drop and she developed a complete cardio-respiratory arrest.

In Jenessa's case her heart muscle was more susceptible to the effects of a low oxygen level. The shunt which had been placed surgically, preferentially, directs blood from the aorta into the pulmonary arteries. When a baby's blood pressure is normal, a balance is maintained between the blood flow to the body and the blood flow to the lungs. However, if there is a rapid change in the blood pressure the lungs may continue to receive additional blood flow through the shunt, which occurs at the expense of the blood supply to the baby's heart muscle. In Jenessa's case her heart muscle was deprived of the necessary blood to maintain normal function. As a result, her heart muscle cells became swollen in response to diminished blood flow. This resulted in a decrease in Jenessa's left ventricular ejection fraction.

As with most organs in the body, the 'healing

process' will occur if the blood supply is restored within a reasonable length of time. In Jenessa's case, the cardiopulmonary resuscitation was instituted promptly and blood flow to the heart muscle was then restored. The main goal during her recovery was to maintain her blood pressure and oxygenation levels in order for the heart to recover and for the swelling in her heart muscle cells to resolve. Jenessa was given a combination of cardiac medications which improved her heart function and at the same time reduced the workload of her heart. (If the heart muscle is dilated it cannot pump blood sufficiently. By reducing the workload on the heart, the heart muscle cells will be able to recover much more quickly.) Jenessa was given intravenous medication referred to as Milrinone. This medication dilates the arteries in the body which in effect reduces the blood pressure and reduces the amount of work that the heart has to perform. This medication also works on the myocardial cells by increasing the influx of calcium which then increases the contractile function of the cells. The Milrinone medication was a lifesaver for Jenessa and allowed her heart function to return to normal over the subsequent 5 days following her respiratory arrest. Despite the significant insult which occurred to Jenessa's heart, her brain did not appear to sustain any permanent damage. We were subsequently able to wean Jenessa off her medications and off the ventilator after approximately six days time, and she was then discharged with her mother four days later.

CHAPTER 8:

THE DREADED G-TUBE

As the days progressed and her heart continued to improve, Dr. King could still find no heart related reason for Jenessa to have stopped breathing in the first place. In conferring with Dr. Cynthia Cristofani, (the Pediatric Intensivist in charge of this particular hospital stay) they decided that the original idea of regurgitating something into her lungs and thus causing her airway to become blocked was the only reasonable explanation.

Again, my head was spinning. It did that a lot! I remembered way back when Jenessa was only a few days old and Georgia had told me about a gastronomy tube, known as a G-tube. She had explained that by having this surgically implanted, we could do away with the NG-tube, and the many difficulties associated with it.

Now, as I sat there in the hospital and listened to the doctors speak of her choking, I wondered if we'd made the wrong decision by not having the G-tube put in months ago.

I had just been so certain that I could 'teach' Jenessa how to eat. I assumed that by feeding her enough bottles, she'd learn to eat/suck well enough to be nourished. But she was already three months old. I was still having to supplement her with tube feedings after most bottle feedings. This required her to have the NG-tube in at all times, and even though I no longer needed Debbie to insert it, I still dreaded having to deal with it.

Dr. King brought up the subject of the G-tube, and I immediately knew there was no longer a choice. The bigger Jenessa got, the more bothersome the NG-tube would become. How would she ever learn to eat right with a tube down her nose? It didn't look good, and it couldn't feel good. Once it was inserted it had to be taped to the skin on her cheek, or else it would come out with any movement. Because of her sensitive skin, it caused a horrible rash on her face. Just as soon as the rash would clear up I'd have to change sides, use more tape on the new side, and hope the other side would clear up before it was time to change it back. Most days one side of her cute little face was spotted with blood, ripped raw by the tape. Not only would the G-tube make feeding her easier and caring for her easier, it might even save her from ever choking again. (Talk about a bonus!) So Bill and I agreed to yet another surgery. My friend Margo was so sad that our baby was going to have more holes put into her.

"Was there any part of Jenessa's body that hadn't been poked, pinched, or cut?", she asked.

Sadly, I answered, "No."

The surgery took place on December 30, with no complications. Finally, for the first time in her life, Jenessa's face would be free of the NG-tube. No tape, no tube, no nothing. Just her beautiful little face, soon to be rash-free.

Here, directly from the doctor's surgical notes, is how the procedure was done:

> --The endoscope was passed without difficulty through the mouth into the cavity of the esophagus. Positioning for placement of a per cutaneous endoscopic gastronomy was determined by a combination of trans illumination and direct pressure. Superficial incision was made in the abdominal skin; through that incision a catheter was placed. A wire was passed through the endoscope. This was looped around the plastic portion of the cannula. Wire was then passed into the stomach. This was grasped with a snare. It was pulled out through the mouth. The wire was then attached to the aft end of the #16 French Pezzer with the inner bolster removed. This pulled down through the mouth and out through the abdominal wall. It was cinched in place to another bolster. The patient handled the procedure well.

The next day Jenessa was extubated without incident. Her overall health continued to improve, slowly but surely. Dr. Cristofani was an incredible anchor of support. It seemed that she never left the hospital; she was there day and night. She provided us with updates and answers and everything else we needed throughout our stay. Just another person we will be forever indebted to. Someone we were honored to spend New Years' Eve with.

Pretty soon Jenessa was rolling over in her crib, pulling her tubes out, and messing with all the wires. As much as this made everyone's job more difficult, we all rejoiced that she was re-gaining her strength and asserting herself. She was soon transferred out of the PICU and into a private pediatric room, where we stayed for two more days. We, yes we, were discharged on January 6, 2000.

It was when I was driving the two of us home that I finally had a meltdown. I started to cry uncontrollably, and had to pull over to the side of the road until the racking sobs subsided. I had been listening to everyone tell me for the last few weeks that the only reason that Jenessa was alive was because I had been able to perform CPR. The nurses and doctors had been amazed that a mother could keep her wits about her under such dire circumstances. They praised my efforts, and high-fived me like some sort of hero.

This was completely ludicrous, as I had only done what needed to be done. My choices were to perform CPR or watch her die; there were no other options. But, the enormity of it didn't hit me until now, when I was on my way home. Two weeks ago Jenessa had been blue and stiff, and now she was cooing in the back seat of my car. I got out and kissed her, and thanked her for not leaving us. Even more importantly, I thanked God for not taking her, and for helping me back on that awful day. I certainly had not done it alone.

CHAPTER 9:

FEBRUARY 6, 2000

Finally, Jenessa seemed healthy. She was getting stronger and more alert, and acting more and more like a "normal" child every day. She was curious about her surroundings, starting to play with toys, and beginning to recognize her siblings. She was learning to eat (suck) better, and there were even days when I didn't have to use the G-tube to supplement her bottle feedings. She looked so much better without the NG-tube taped to her face, and her skin cleared up without it. And of course, she got cuter with each passing day!

It was early February when Pastor Terry O'Casey, from our church, came by to ask me a favor. He wanted me to speak at church on Sunday, to the entire congregation. His sermon was to be titled "Why bad things happen to good people" and he thought my testimony would be inspiring.

I was in a panic. I was not a public speaker, and was uncomfortable at the thought of being put in the limelight. I had no idea what I was going to do. How could I say no to a man who had been praying for me and my family for months and months? How could I say no to a man who miraculously showed up in the Emergency Room whenever Jenessa had been there?

Pastor Terry sensed my uneasiness, or lets be honest about it, my panic! He assured me that I could do this. What did he know? I was a wreck, an absolute nervous wreck. I agreed to do it anyway, as I couldn't figure any way out.

A few days later, after giving his sermon, Pastor Terry called me up to the pulpit. I nervously shared the condensed version of Jenessa's life, and how God had helped me and my family through desperate times. I spoke about being given the option to abort her, and instead how Bill and I felt so honored to have been chosen by God to be her parents. Then my friend Debbie brought Jenessa up to me, and I could see people begin to tear up, as she was still so small and fragile.

It was overwhelming; I watched as Jenessa touched those people's lives on that day. I watched as the entire congregation applauded her existence. And then, I watched as seven people came forward and accepted Jesus into their hearts. It wasn't my speech, which had lasted less than ten minutes. It was Jenessa.

CHAPTER 10:

FEBRUARY THROUGH SEPTEMBER

Jenessa continued to grow stronger. She went to Jackie's basketball games and softball games. She went on family outings, laughed when Justin threw her up into the air, and watched every move Jessi made. She became a regular part of our family, and days would go by without any talk of heart defects or Down syndrome. In fact, it would take a doctors appointment or therapy session for Bill and I to be reminded that she even had Down syndrome. It was no longer something we focused on. We focused on her, not her syndrome. We focused on our little girl.

So many people choose instead to focus on the syndrome. We have a friend with a disabled son, and she constantly blames his disability for all of his shortcomings. If her son is mean, it's because of his disability. If her son breaks out in a rash, it's because of his disability. If her son hits another child at school, it's because of his disability.

Bill and I have tried to get her to look at him as a little boy, but she can't see past his disability. All she can see is his affliction. She doesn't see the incredible person her son would become if only she'd stop enabling him.

***

I want to share with you a bit about our daughter's name. All of our children's names begin with J, so hers had to as well. My friend Denise suggested early in my pregnancy that we name her something different, so there would never be a question as to which child was being referred to. In other words, she suggested we not name her something common like Jane. Not because it isn't a beautiful name, but because that way no one could ever have the following conversation:

"Did you see Jane today?"

"Which Jane do you mean?"

"You know, the Jane with Down syndrome."

By naming her something out of the ordinary, we could hopefully avoid her ever being referred to as "the one with Down syndrome". Besides, there's nothing ordinary about her.

One of the most frustrating things about having a child with special needs is dealing with ignorant people. When I meet new people or I see old friends, they often tell me how sorry they feel for me, or how sorry they are that Jenessa was born with Down syndrome. When I tell them I'm not sorry, they think I'm in denial. But I'm not! I wouldn't want her any other way. I have no idea why people can't understand that.

Another problem I face is that people often categorize Down children. Do you know how often I hear:

"Down children are so loving...blah,blah,blah."

"Down children don't have a mean bone in their bodies...blah,blah,blah."

"At least Down kids are sweet, even if they aren't smart"

HELLO!! Not all Down children are kind. Not all blondes have more fun. The grass isn't always greener on the other side. No person with a disability should be thought of in any light other than that of their own person. People who have pre-conceived notions of how a person will behave or will not behave, based on that person's disability, need to get a grip on reality. Just because Jenessa has Down syndrome does not mean that she's retarded, loving, slow, or kind. *Jenessa is Jenessa.* Just like any other child. She has her own personality. She has her own likes and dislikes. Just because a child is deaf does not mean they're dumb. Just because a child is born without a leg doesn't mean they won't learn to walk. Just because Jenessa has Down syndrome does not guarantee that she will grow up to be sweet and loving. That's up to us, as her parents, to instill in her. Just like it is with our other three children.

CHAPTER 11:

THE BIG ONE

As Jenessa's first birthday drew closer, we all knew that it was almost time for her second, and hopefully last, open heart surgery.

Dr. King decided she was ready. She was healthy, strong, happy, and a little over fourteen pounds. I remember her sitting on the examining table in Dr. King's office shaking her head as he started her routine exam. She pulled off each wire he attached to her chest in hopes of doing an EEG. She moved his hand as he tried to do an echocardiogram of her heart. She gave him nothing but trouble, and smiled at him while he pleaded with her to be still. He smiled back.

Next he scheduled an appointment to do a cardiac catheterization, which is a test that offers clear, accurate information about the heart. During the test, which is performed in the hospital under general anesthesia, a thin tube called a catheter is fed through a blood vessel. It was inserted through a small cut made by Dr. King in her groin, then guided through the blood vessel all the way up to her heart. Dr. King tracked the course of the catheter by watching it on a special viewing screen. A variety of measurements can be performed while the catheter is in place, and then the catheter is removed. In Jenessa's case, Dr. King used the data gleaned from the procedure to make a sort of 'road map' of Jenessa's anatomy. This would help the surgeons better plan for her upcoming surgery.

Next we met with Dr. Albert Starr, who along with Dr. John Iguidbashian, would perform the surgery. I had heard so much about Dr. Starr, about his history of accomplishments, breakthroughs, and his invention of what is now known as the Starr valve. He is a legend in the cardiac community. As Dr. King put it, "...[he is]the most detailed surgeon on the planet." I was concerned a bit because of his age, I think he was 74 at the time of her surgery, but Dr. King, who I trust implicitly, assured me that Dr. Starr was the doctor I wanted. I later learned that patients fly in from all over the United States just to have Dr. Starr perform their operations. How lucky we were to have him in our own back yard.

The meeting was terribly frightening. We met in a large, ornately decorated conference room, where Dr. Starr explained the intricacies of the surgery to us. Actually, he explained it to Bill, as these were the details I refused to allow my brain to comprehend. He did get my attention, however, when he told us the fatality rate for this type of surgery was 10%. That seemed awfully high to me, and it scared me to death. He felt confident there would be no problems, but of course, wanted to be clear that there were no guarantees. This brilliant man was telling us the truth, but it was a truth neither one of us wanted to hear. He would operate, attempt to repair our daughter's heart, and probably, most likely, succeed. But what if he didn't? What if Jenessa became part of that 10% statistic?

We left with pictures, diagrams, and more cardiac handouts than I would ever read. Bill, of course, read them all. Not only did he read them, but he completely understood them. We went home and hugged our baby, knowing that in less than two weeks we would be entrusting her entire future to a man we'd just met.

Next I had an appointment to give blood. I wanted to have blood ready in case Jenessa ran into trouble during surgery and needed a transfusion. I remember being so happy the morning of my appointment, because I finally felt like I was contributing something. Before they took my blood they ran some routine tests, to make sure my blood was healthy and would be "useable". You can imagine my surprise, when the tests showed I was anemic. Thus, I would not be a suitable donor.

This had a profound effect on me, and I don't know if I can even put my feelings into words. I felt like a terrible mother, who could not provide my daughter with something so basic, yet incredibly important. The nurse tried to reassure me, but I was not consolable. I hadn't been taking care of myself, hadn't been eating right, hadn't had enough sleep. I was so concentrated on Jenessa, and what she was about to go through. I was busy trying to hide my own fears from Justin, Jackie, and Jessi. I did the laundry, cooked the meals, kept the house clean, and I made sure my family was well taken care of. I wanted their lives to seem as normal as possible. I wanted my life to seem as normal as possible. I was so busy going through the motions, so busy trying to be Super-mom, and now I couldn't even donate my own blood, because I was running on empty. I was completely and totally devastated.

Bill, the rock that he is, stepped up and filled in. There were no available appointments for him to give blood at this late date, but the nurse, bless her heart, agreed to stay late to accommodate him.

So Bill gave blood later that day. I stayed home and pretended, once again, to be Super-mom. I wore my bravest face, and acted like everything was okay. I wasn't sure how much longer I could keep up the charade.

Finally, it was the day before surgery. We brought Jenessa to the hospital so they could do blood work and run the necessary pre-surgery tests. We did enough paperwork to fill a file cabinet.

We checked into a room at the Ronald McDonald House across the street. We bathed Jenessa in a special disinfectant soap, as instructed by the doctors. We ate a little dinner, and then took Jenessa to the playroom. She sat there playing with all the toys. She hummed in the toy car, turning the keys and pretending to drive. Bill and I watched, knowing full well what tomorrow would bring. We would take our baby, who was not in any duress, back to the hospital for surgery. Somehow, it was easier to face surgery when your child was sick. Jenessa seemed perfectly healthy. But Dr. King assured us that is was much easier to operate on Jenessa now, while she was nice and strong. If we waited for her heart to give out, her chances of survival would decrease dramatically. This made perfect sense to the intellectual side of our brains, but it was hard emotionally to watch her playing and laughing, knowing that tomorrow she'd be laying on a steel table.

CHAPTER 12:

OCTOBER 17, 2000

We brought Jenessa to the hospital at 5:30a.m. She was admitted, fitted with a bright green ID bracelet, and sent to a private room to wait. When the time came, we were allowed to go down to the operating room with her. There the anesthesiologist briefed us, and then Dr. King miraculously appeared, as usual, to answer any last minute questions. And then she was gone. Just like that. A moment later a nurse came out.

"I know this is going to be one of the hardest days of your life. But it should comfort you to know that this is what these doctors do, day in and day out. It's just a regular work day for them, and they know what they're doing."

It really was comforting, in a strange way, to think of it like that. Bill and I were then sent to the waiting room, where we prepared to spend the day. We knew that the surgery could take up to eight hours, and when you figure in prep time and recovery time, we knew we wouldn't see Jenessa again for quite a while. It was going to be a very long day.

Somehow, some way, probably by the grace of God, I wasn't a nervous wreck. I actually felt relief that this day was finally here. Growing Jenessa bigger, and getting Jenessa healthier this past year, had all led up to this day. It was like this big surgery cloud had been hovering over all of us, and today it had burst wide open.

A couple of hours later, we were surprised to see our friends Mike and Eva Hague. We didn't know they were coming, but their visit helped entertain us during the long wait.

Their story of how they got to the hospital was priceless. For some reason they had it in their minds that Jenessa was being operated on at a different hospital up the road. When they got there, they were told they had no patient there named Jenessa. Apparently Mike and Eva put up quite an argument, insisting that she was there. When they were finally convinced she wasn't, they made some calls, and went to another hospital, only to be turned away again. They visited three or four hospitals before finally tracking us down, getting lost numerous times along the way. Listening to them talk about getting directions from strangers, making wrong turns, and visiting hospitals they never knew existed, was hysterical. Their morning mishaps made for great storytelling, which was exactly what we needed to get our minds off of the surgery. I much preferred thinking about them driving all over town than Jenessa being hooked up to the heart lung machine downstairs. They even managed to drag us off to the cafeteria, where I surprised everyone by actually eating. We'd been getting periodic updates from the O.R., where everything was progressing as planned. With each bit of good news, I became more and more relaxed.

After lunch we made our way back to the waiting room, and settled in for the home stretch. Mike and Eva stayed with us and prayed with us, and kept us busy talking about anything and everything, except what was happening downstairs.

Finally, Dr. Starr blew into the room. He wiped sweat from his brow, and managed to flop down into a chair. He was mentally and physically exhausted. The first words out of his mouth are words I'll never forget.

"Your daughter no longer has a heart defect."

Then the flood gates opened. I was crying so hard I almost didn't hear what he said next:

"We were able to do a complete repair of her heart."

He went on to explain how they repaired each defect, what materials they used, and how happy he was with the outcome. Pretty soon all I was hearing was BLAH... BLAH... BLAH... BLAH... BLAH. I knew Bill would listen, and comprehend, all the medical details as Dr. Starr explained them. All I could hear was, your daughter no longer has a heart defect, your daughter no longer has a heart defect. Those were the only words I needed. They've become my eight favorite words in the English language.

It turned out, however, that there was a bit of bad news. Jenessa was currently using a temporary pacemaker, hooked up on the outside of her body. Apparently, with all the delicate maneuvering of her heart during the surgery, the circuit that is supposed to send messages from the top chamber of the heart to the bottom wasn't working. Dr. Starr was hopeful that this was only a temporary setback, and when the swelling went down everything would start to function properly again. He assured us it was not life threatening, and would not impact her quality of life. We would just have to wait and see.

When Dr. Starr left we prayed again, thanking God for watching over our baby and her doctors. Mike and Eva left, and we waited another hour while the nurses in the PICU attended to Jenessa's post surgery needs. When she was finally stable, we were allowed in to see her.

She looked like the Pillsbury Dough-Boy, under a pile of wires and tubes and buzzing machines. She was *so* puffy. Her chest was bulging and red, with dried blood outlining her freshly made scar. She was of course intubated, and the ventilator was helping her breathe. When I glanced at the monitors, I almost fainted. Her oxygen saturations fluctuated between 99 and 100, the same way as people without heart defects. For some reason I hadn't been expecting this. I knew they had fixed her heart, but I didn't realize it would be working normally, pumping normally, and beating normally. It was!

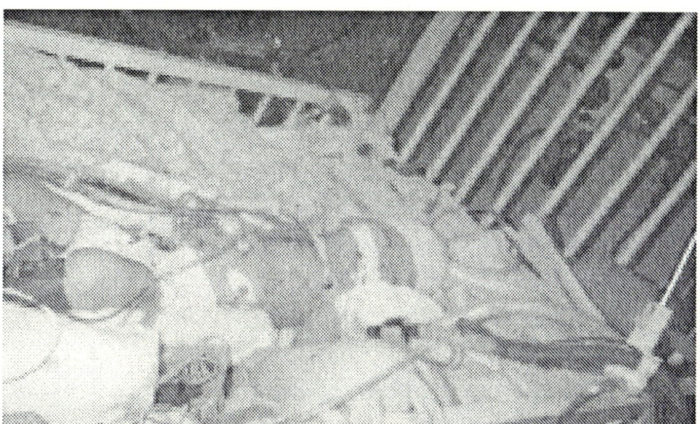

The rest of the day was mostly uneventful, which, from a surgical point of view, is exactly the way you want it. She slept, we watched; so far–so good.

The next morning Jenessa was feeling more like herself, and she decided she didn't want the breathing tube down her throat. So, like a typical one year old, she tried to pull it out. She was so uncomfortable that she started to thrash about, grabbing the intubation tube and pulling– hard. In doing so she punctured a hole in her lung, and the machines went haywire. Doctors and nurses filled her room, and we were asked to leave.

They ended up having to insert a chest tube, which would allow her lung to re-inflate. Just one more hole into her precious little body. Then they sedated her big time, giving her enough meds to pretty much knock her out for the next few days. They even tied her little hands down, as they didn't want any more complications caused by her being uncomfortable. As scary as all of this was, I was secretly proud of my daughter for once again asserting her independence. I'd just prefer she not cause any more harm to herself in doing so.

Jenessa was extubated two days later without incident. The rest of her stay was pretty much textbook, with most of my time spent watching the monitors, in hopes they would show some sign that her atrium, the upper chamber of her heart, was talking to her ventricle, the lower chamber of her heart. Unfortunately, this was not going to be the case. She never did come out of her 'heart block'.

Finally, after almost two weeks of waiting and hoping, the doctors decided it was time to 'install' a pacemaker. This would monitor her heart and make sure that the atrium delivered messages to the ventricle. Her atrium was beating on its own and sending the signals, they just weren't reaching the ventricle because the circuitry had been damaged.

> The "natural" pacemaker of the heart is called the sinus node. The sinus node is a small mass of special cells in the top of the right atrium of the heart. It produces the electrical impulse that goes to the left atrium and travels down to reach the ventricular

> muscle. These impulses cause the heart to contract, or beat. The term artificial pacemaker refers to an electrical device that is used to replace a defective natural pacemaker or conduction pathway. The artificial pacemaker controls the heart's beating and rhythm by emitting a series of electrical discharges.

When my husbands curiosity got the best of him , he asked the doctors how much a pacemaker was going to cost. Not because it would make any difference, as we would have done anything or paid anything to keep Jenessa alive. Not to mention, we had long since satisfied the deductible on our insurance! He was simply curious.

"About ten thousand dollars, installed." The doctor's answered.

Everyone in the room broke out laughing. The kind of laughter that comes from deep within; the kind that releases stress and tension. I mean, what else could we do, but laugh?

"Installed?" Bill asked. "What is it, a pacemaker or a car part?"

We knew the doctors well enough to know they weren't being heartless, rude, or insensitive. It was simply the easiest way to explain the true cost, which would include the part, the pacemaker; and the labor, the surgery. So she was taken, yet again, into surgery. The permanent pacemaker was inserted into Jenessa's upper right abdomen, and finally, they were able to completely sew her up. No more wires hanging out of her chest. No more open wounds. Just another scar, covering a machine that will remain with Jenessa for the rest of her life.

As time goes by, the pacemaker batteries will have to be replaced. We're told, because her usage levels will be low, that the current batteries should last about six years. At that time she'll have to have a quick surgery, which should keep her in the hospital only over one night. Then, when she hits her late teens or early twenties, the doctors will actually replace the pacemaker, and move it to the upper left quadrant of her chest. But we'll deal with all that when the time comes. For now, we just wanted to get Jenessa well, so we could take her home.

Here, in Dr. King's own words, are the details of her surgery:

> Over the proceeding six months, Jenessa's growth and development had been satisfactory. In addition, her echocardiograms had revealed growth of both her pulmonary arteries and her pulmonary valves. Consequently, we decided that she had reached the size where she could safely undergo a complete repair of her defect. Jenessa's complete repair did require use of a heart-lung bypass machine. Her chest was opened through the previous incision which we used for her shunt procedure.
>
> Once the chest was opened the heart was exposed and she had three tubes placed in her heart; two in the veins draining the blood from the body, and one from the aorta. Jenessa's blood flow was then diverted into the heart-lung machine where carbon dioxide was removed and oxygen was added. The oxygenated blood was returned to the body through the tube in the aorta. Dr. Albert Starr, Jenessa's attending cardiac surgeon then opened the right atrium and a piece of Dacron was utilized to close the hole between the two pumping chambers (ie the ventricular septal defects: VSD.) The common AV valve was then reconstructed to form a relatively normal two leaflet mitral valve and a three leaflet tricuspid valve. The valve tissue was then attached to the VSD patch. In Jenessa's case her VSD extended somewhat more anteriorly and the patch had to be extended toward the aortic root. Once the VSD was closed the atrial septal defect (ASD) was closed with a piece of Jenessa's own tissue. A piece of pericardium, which is the normal tissue which surrounds the heart, was utilized to close the ASD.

Once the holes were closed an incision was made on the right ventricular muscle below the pulmonary valve in order to enlarge the pathway from the right ventricle to the pulmonary valve. A small piece of pericardium was utilized to enlarge this pathway. Finally, a small patch was placed on the main pulmonary artery to enlarge the pathway between the pulmonary valve and the pulmonary arteries. Jenessa was on the heart-lung machine for approximately 2.5 hours. She was then weaned off the bypass circuit and her own heart muscle resumed pumping.

Unfortunately, her heart rate was slower than normal and we discovered that her conduction system had been injured during the procedure. Normally, impulses from the sinus node will conduct through the atrio-ventricular node into the right ventricle. In Jenessa's case the atrio-ventricular node was injured during the repair of the ventricular septal defect. As a result, the impulses from the sinus node were unable to effectively stimulate the conduction pathways in the ventricles. Her heart was initially paced with an external pacemaker. After ten days time it was clear that her rhythm was not going to return to normal, and at that time a decision was made to proceed with placement of a permanent pacemaker. Jenessa then returned to the operating room where a dual chamber permanent pacemaker was placed. An incision was then made at the lower end of the previous incision and the sternum was once again opened. A pacing lead was attached to the right atrium and a second lead was attached to the right ventricle. These leads were then attached to a permanent pacemaker and the pacemaker was then implanted into a pocket that was created below the abdominal muscle. This permanent pacemaker then took over for the temporary pacemaker which had been utilized for the past ten days. The pacemaker was implanted without problems. Jenessa returned once again to the Pediatric Intensive Care Unit where she was once again weaned off the ventilator. She then returned to the pediatrics ward after another 24 hours in the ICU.

Douglas H. King, MD
Children's Cardiac Center of Oregon

****

The day after the pacemaker was implanted, we were moved out of the PICU into a regular pediatric room. By now Jenessa was sitting up, playing with toys, looking through books, watching cartoons, and eating normally. Two days later, after sixteen days in the hospital, Bill came to get us and take us home. Except for routine check-ups, we haven't been back.

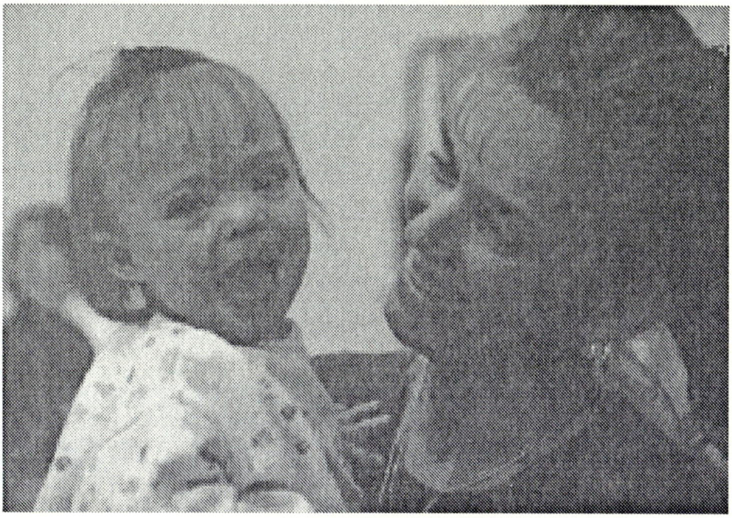

CHAPTER 13:

POST SURGERY LIFE

We visit Dr. King every three months, mostly to check on Jenessa's pacemaker settings, also, to reassure me that she's fine. I'm the one who needs Dr. King to reconfirm that everything is okay. It is!

Within a few months Jenessa learned to crawl, and began to communicate using simple signs. The experts now believe that sign language actually helps kids learn to verbalize sooner. Her first signs were: "more", "me", "help", "eat", "thank you", and "love you"; her first "real" words were "bye-bye" (pronounced 'buh-bye'). All of these were accompanied by enthusiastic waving and happy smiles.

In December, less than three months after her surgery, Bill and I removed Jenessa's G-tube. We were scheduled to bring her to the hospital on a Monday, but on Saturday the tube started to leak. We paged the doctor, and instead of driving two hours to his office through a terrible rainstorm, he walked us through the removal steps over the phone. Bill did the actual removal, while I relayed the information from the doctor. Most people cringe when I tell them we did this ourselves. But after everything we'd been through, it was really no big deal. We've really come a long way. A few years ago there was no way I would have even considered -not- going to the doctor's office. No way!

Christmas was more special than ever before. We were so, very, grateful for all that we had been blessed with. The next year brought many milestones, as Jenessa learned to walk, then run. Although she wasn't very verbal, she had superb comprehension of the English language. She understood everything we said, and she followed our directions with great enthusiasm and joy. If only our other children behaved so well! She brought us books to read as she crawled up onto our laps. She fell in love with Veggie Tales. She loved the swing set, and climbing all over our furniture. Her favorite thing to do was cook with me in the kitchen, or 'pretend cook' in her own toy kitchen. She also loved doing any sort of chore, because she so much wanted to 'help mommy' like her older siblings. Sorting the Tupperware, putting away groceries, and re-stocking the toilet paper filled her with pride.

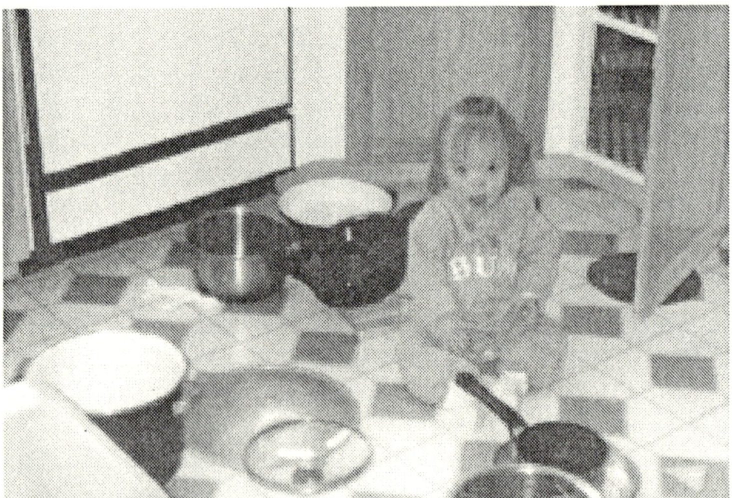

If all of this is sounding pretty 'normal' to you, then you're getting my point. We'd been through some medical nightmares, some very scary times, but we'd made it. And now we could sit back and enjoy watching our daughter grow up, just like any other child.

Oops! I almost forgot. Jenessa has Down syndrome. I'm reminded whenever she has a therapy session or doctor's appointment. But only then. Mostly, she's just a regular part of our family. We don't treat her any differently than our other children. We don't make excuses or exceptions for her. She has no idea that the world has classified her as disabled. We certainly haven't. Differently 'abled' maybe, but disabled, never!

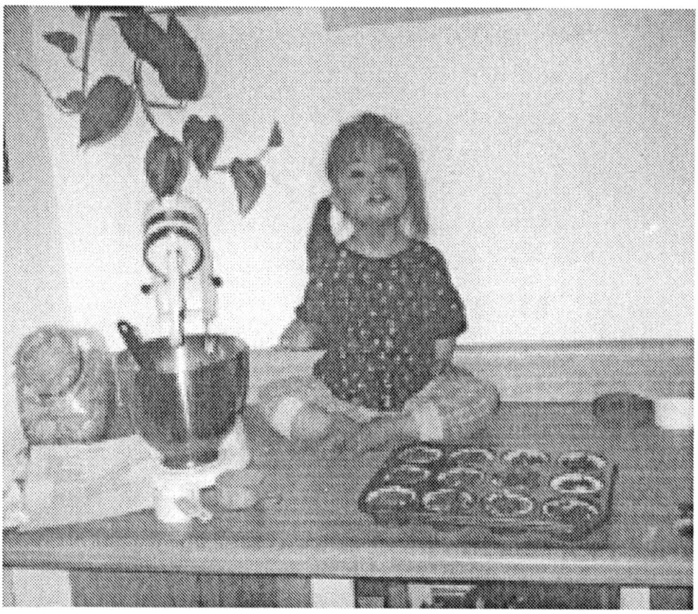

Baking Muffins with Mom

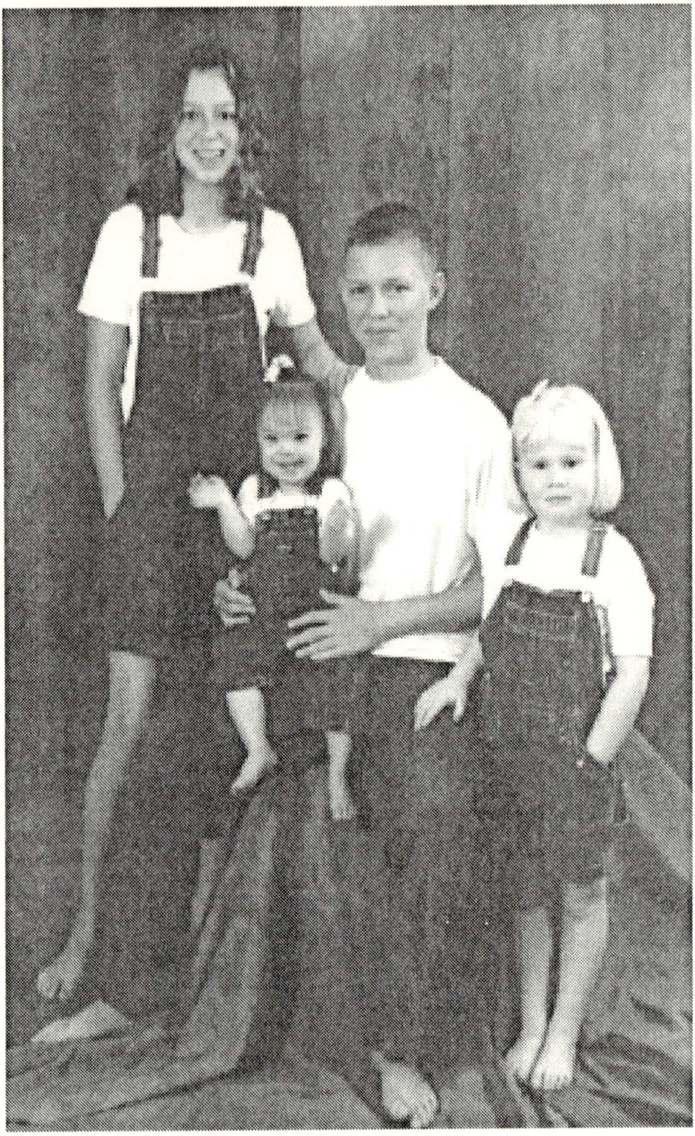

Justin, Jackie, Jessi, and Jenessa: June 2001

CHAPTER 14:

DOCTORS, THERAPISTS, AND BOOKS, OH MY!

During the first three years of Jenessa's life, we have been very blessed with incredible doctors, wonderful nurses, and highly educated therapists. I've read some powerful and informative books. These people and these books are the reason Jenessa is alive today, and the reason why she is doing well. However, there's always a spoiler in every group.

Our first bad experience came in the form of our local pediatrician. I'll call her Dr. Dumb.

I've already told you about her view on the nutritional supplements we were giving Jenessa. She had equally negative views about her getting a G-tube. She told me it was completely unnecessary, and could not possibly help because now Jenessa would never learn to eat 'normal'. She knew about the choking incident, and how Jenessa had nearly died because of it. She knew about her trouble gaining weight, and how this was of critical importance in determining when she could have her pending surgery. But most of all, she knew I was not the type of mother who would use the G-tube in lieu of bottle feeding. I explained to her that I was using it during the day only as a back-up, and nightly for her drip feedings. I can't imagine how Jenessa would have ever been able to eat enough to gain weight without those nightly feedings, but Dr. Dumb just rolled her eyes. She was not at all supportive on this issue.

Another time, during a routine physical, she told me how Down kids always have a lot of ear problems. She said we should schedule an appointment soon for her to have tubes surgically put in, as this would alleviate all the future infections she was sure to have.

I reminded her that Jenessa had never had an ear infection. Not one, not ever. She replied by saying that it was only a matter of time, and I needed to face up to the necessity of tubes. I told her that I wouldn't even consider it until she's had enough infections for it to be deemed necessary.

Last year Jessi, my middle daughter, was having trouble hearing, and a specialist found she had tremendous fluid built up in her ear canals. To make a long story short, Jessi had tubes put in both ears. At her post-surgery follow up appointment, I asked the specialist about Jenessa's ears. She said it was quite common for Down kids to require tubes, which I knew from all my reading, but it was certainly not an absolute. She didn't put tubes in just because a child had Down syndrome, and she was shocked by Dr. Dumb's pre-mature suggestion for surgery.

She took a look in Jenessa's ears, and found her to have the typically small ear canals commonly associated with Down Syndrome. There was a large build up of wax, but no infection or drainage. Using a really small instrument, this doctor was able to remove the wax while I held Jenessa, right there in her office. The whole procedure took less than ten minutes, and Jenessa didn't even cry. And to this day, Jenessa has not required tubes be put in her ears. She has yet to have an ear infection.

The final straw came the time when Jenessa broke out in a rash from head to toe. She was covered in these small, pin sized red dots, on every inch of her tiny body. I took her to see Dr. Dumb, who immediately diagnosed her as having meningococcal disease. Now I'm just a mother, with no medical schooling whatsoever, but I knew this wasn't meningococcal disease, or anything in that 'family' of diseases. I had seen this terrible disease during my times at the hospital, and knew that it meant loss of limbs, and often loss of life. I also knew that at the onset the patient developed a big blotchy rash, usually dark purple in color. Not small, pin sized red dots. I mentioned this to the doctor, who told me she knew meningococcal when she saw it. She also reminded me that I wasn't a doctor, so I shouldn't question her expertise. She wanted to rush Jenessa to the hospital, and have IV antibiotics started immediately.

Just then, Dr. Dumb's partner walked into the examining room. First thing out of her mouth was to ask if Jenessa had recently had the MMR (measles, mumps, and rubella) vaccine. I answered yes, and calculated that she'd had it ten days ago.

"She has the measles," she told me. She explained that there is always a chance of contracting the disease you're being vaccinated against, and that was obviously what had happened. A big, nasty shot of antibiotics in each thigh and we were on our way.

The next morning the spots were mostly gone, and Jenessa was feeling good as new. I never went back to see Dr. Dumb again. I wanted a doctor who would diagnose my daughter, not her disability. Then there was the Speech Therapist from hell.

We were initially, sent through our county's Early Intervention Program, a Speech Therapist who I'll call Cindy. Cindy is a middle aged woman who was constantly surprised by Jenessa's progress.

When I first met with Cindy, Jenessa was just a few months old. Cindy listed a number of things that Jenessa would never do, and set up some feeding goals that she considered reasonable for a child with Down syndrome. One of the first goals she established was to get Jenessa to suck on her bottle, the nipple, without her tongue protruding. When I told her that wasn't a problem and Jenessa didn't do that, she asked me to prove it to her by feeding Jenessa while she watched. I was happy to oblige, as it ticked me off that she didn't believe me, and was making negative assumptions about my daughter. After seeing Jenessa eat, she was amazed that a baby with Down syndrome could nipple correctly, without a protruding tongue.

Over the next year or so, we had many similar incidents. Cindy would tell me what Jenessa couldn't do, what she would never be able to do, and I would set out to prove her wrong. It became my mission to prove her wrong, and in doing so, I hoped I could change her dated perceptions about Down syndrome. I talked candidly with her about her attitude, and asked her to please try to look at Jenessa as an individual, with individual problems; but all she could see was the syndrome.

My argument was, and still is, that Jenessa is a little girl *first* who happens to have Down syndrome. She also happens to have brown hair and brown eyes, an infectious laugh and a beautiful smile. I believe that she would, could, and will do everything a "normal" child can do. It will take her longer, and she'll have to work harder, but she'll get there. Cindy couldn't see past the Down syndrome; she couldn't look at the little girl. I finally told Cindy that I'd had enough, and I wouldn't listen to her negative assumptions and ideas any more. I told her not to call me or ever try to see Jenessa again.

Lucky for me, a new Speech Therapist had recently come to work in our county, and she was sent to replace Cindy. At the time, I was willing to go outside the community and hire my own; but Kate is awesome! She looks at Jenessa like I do, as an individual. She took the time to watch Jenessa and to learn about her capabilities and deficiencies before setting any goals for her. Imagine that.

This proves that you, the parent, will be your child's biggest advocate. If you settle for a bad therapist, your child will pay the price. If you settle for an incompetent doctor, your child could face unnecessary treatment and/or surgeries. Ask questions! Learn whatever it takes! Stand up for your child! No one else is going to.

And whatever you do, don't believe everything you read.

Back when I first found out that my baby would be born with Down syndrome, I picked up a book I'd been reading before I knew. I looked up Down syndrome in the index, and read the various pages that dealt with it. The author refers to Down syndrome in a completely negative way, and speaks about the different tests that can be done to "eliminate this worry from your itinerary".

How many women had read these passages, and aborted their pregnancies because of it? The author goes on to talk about a friend of hers who had an amniocentesis done to determine if her unborn baby had Down syndrome, and "how all their lives were shortened by the worrisome wait" (for the results), and how thankful they all were to find out the baby would be "normal".

I was disgusted by her cavalier attitude, appalled that she could write about genetic abnormalities in such a way, and even worse, actually have her stupidity published. Not only was she ignorant beyond words, but it actually saddened me that there were people out there who felt so threatened by a child with special needs. So many people just don't get it. They just can't understand, because their hearts are cold and closed. How sad for them.

So watch what you read. Just because it's in print doesn't mean it's true. And more than anything, be open to new ideas of what is normal, and what is good. A disabled child is still a child. And all children deserve a chance at a good life. All it takes is a dedicated parent, who becomes a dedicated advocate, looking out for the best interests of his or her very special child.

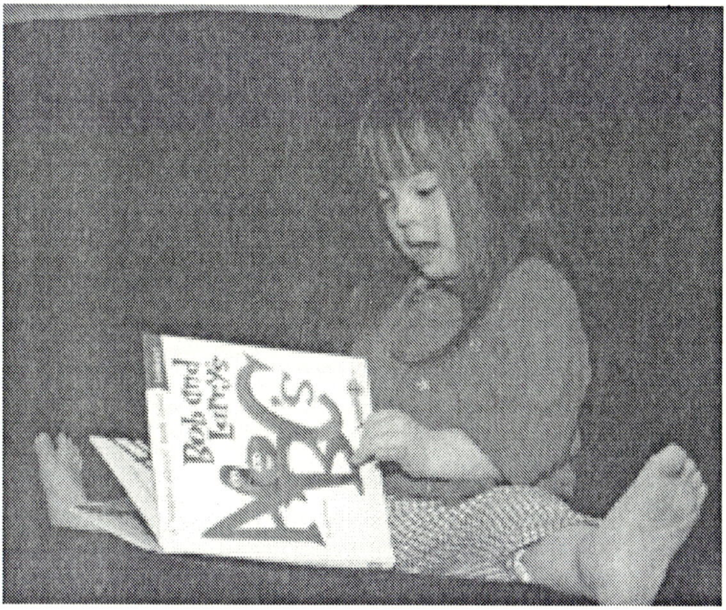

CHAPTER 15:

A NUTRITIONAL ODYSSEY

Early on I discussed the vitamin supplements that Jenessa is taking. What I haven't told you, is that Jenessa is hardly ever sick. I've read so much about poor immune systems being associated with Down syndrome. Ear infections, colds, flus, and respiratory problems are usually commonplace. But not with Jenessa. We joke that while she's had two open heart surgeries, she rarely has a simple cold! *We try to keep our sense of humor.* I have to assume it's because of the Nutrivene, as there is no other explanation.

Some friends of ours have a child with Down syndrome, who is constantly sick. She's been hospitalized numerous times for one infection or another, and has had to have more than one surgery postponed because she was too sick to handle it. Recently she became so ill that she is now receiving antibiotics intravenously at home. While I realize that some children are more susceptible to illness than others, I don't understand why her parents won't at least try these vitamins. They know how healthy Jenessa is; they've seen her energy. But they insist that Jenessa was just born with a stronger immune system than most Down children. While this may in fact be true, I have to think that supplements developed specifically for Down metabolism have to be helping. Most of us take some sort of vitamins ourselves, and the one I take is formulated especially for women. My husband takes one specifically formulated for men. So it only makes sense to me to give Jenessa one specifically formulated for her. Because Down children are often so sick, they fall even further behind developmentally, physically, emotionally, and intellectually. Keeping Jenessa healthy helps her to avoid these setbacks..

Another friend of mine told me she had watched a television show about a mother who was giving her daughter these same vitamins in hopes of changing her daughter's facial characteristics. She was supposedly hoping to make her daughter look more 'normal' and less like a child with Down syndrome. While I have no idea if this is true or not, I can tell you with absolute certainty that this is not my goal. I have no desire to change the way Jenessa looks. I have no desire to change who Jenessa is. My only hope is to boost her immune system, and provide her brain and her heart with the necessary nutrients for optimum health and development. It's as simple as that, with no hidden agenda whatsoever.

In an effort to explain more about nutritional intervention for persons with Down syndrome, I've asked two nationally recognized experts* to help me out. The following is the chapter that they have written specifically for this book.

A chapter dedicated to:

Diet and Nutritional Supplementation in Down syndrome

A Nutritional Odyssey

Co-authors:

Croom, James Jr., Ph.D., FACN
Professor of Nutrition
North Carolina State University 27695

Leichtman, Lawrence G. , MD., Ph.D., FAAP, FACMG
Genetics and Disabilities Diagnostic Care Center
Virginia Beach, Virginia 23454

> "The relation of vitamins to mental disease became evident as soon as vitamins were discovered".
>
> Linus Pauling[1]

[1] Pauling, Linus
Winner of the Nobel Prize in Chemistry (1954)
Winner of the Nobel Peace Prize (1962)

Dedication:

This chapter is dedicated in loving memory of Rachael Mayo, artist and writer, age 19, of Winona, Minnesota, who succumbed, March 1, 2003 at 10:30 am, to the ravages of Hodgkin's disease during the preparation of this manuscript.

To the happy children of
the future,
The children of the past
send greetings.

****

Inscription on the Alma Mater statue by Lorado Taft
University of Illinois at Urbana-Champaign

*Dr. Croom received his Ph.D. in Nutritional Sciences from the Division of Nutritional Sciences at the University of Illinois at Urbana-Champaign, in 1977. He has been at NCSU for 25 years as a research nutritionist; and teaches both undergraduate and graduate courses in comparative nutrition and gastrointestinal physiology. His specialty is Intermediary Metabolism, and he has a subspecialty in Gastrointestinal Physiology. He has published over 200 peer reviewed scientific papers, book chapters, and abstracts in nutritional biochemistry and physiology. He is an internationally recognized expert on gastrointestinal regulation. He holds 5 patents for therapeutic drugs that enhance digestion and absorption of nutrients in humans and animals, the release of growth hormone in humans and animals, and a treatment for Alzheimer's disease. He has given numerous invited lectures in the US, Canada, England, Scotland, Australia, New Zealand, and Indonesia on a variety of nutritional and gastrointestinal topics. He has been a Visiting Associate Professor of Internal Medicine, Division of Gastroenterology at Duke University Medical Center. He is a Fellow of the American College of Nutrition and a Registered Professional Animal Scientist. Memberships in honor societies include Alpha Zeta (Agricultural Honorary), Gamma Sigma Delta (Agricultural Honorary) and Sigma XI (Science Honorary).

*Dr. Leichtman has over 20 years experience in Clinical Genetics. He is on the state and local board (in Virginia) of Directors of the March of Dimes. He is the President of the Board of Directors, Trisomy-21 Research Foundation, Inc. He is a Fellow of the American College of Medical Genetics and a Fellow of the American Academy of Pediatrics. He is the former division director of Genetics at one of the east coast's most prominent medical schools. He currently specializes in clinical genetic evaluations for children and adults, DNA testing for genetic disorders, genetic counseling, behavioral and medical management of the disabled, diagnosis and treatment of metabolic disorders, Targeted Nutritional Intervention for Genetic Disorders, and the treatment of Autism.

Enough said!

Introduction:

Ever since the first professional description of Down syndrome by physician John Langdon Down in 1866, an effective treatment of this disorder has eluded physicians and scientists. The cause of Down syndrome was not determined for over 90 years. It was the discovery of the structure of the cellular basis for inheritance, DNA, by Watson and Crick[2] in 1953, followed by the observation in 1959, by Jerome Lejeune, that persons with Down syndrome contained an extra chromosome in the nucleus of their cells, that some hope of treating this genetic disorder emerged. Still, since the science of molecular biology was in its infancy in the 1950's, this information did not prove immediately useful in developing a treatment for this condition.

Early in the 1940's physician Henry Turkel began attempts to treat the many physical ailments associated with Down syndrome by the administration of increased amounts of vitamins and minerals. His approach was based strictly on intuition since a full appreciation, by the scientific and medical communities, of the importance of the relationship between DNA, chromosomes, genes and the occurrence of Down syndrome was over a decade away. Turkel's regime of vitamins and minerals, named the "U Series" was controversial from the start. His efforts were lauded as successful by many and criticized as scientific quackery by others. This debate continues to this day and now involves newer versions of this vitamin supplementation regime, the most popular of which is called "Targeted Nutritional Intervention" or TNI. What many critics of Turkel's work do not realize was that his approach was well within the accepted limits of the scientific knowledge of his time.

I. Vitamins, Disease and History

The first reported use of a vitamin containing substance to treat a disease was the use of citrus juices (with a high vitamin C content) to cure scurvy (severe deficiency of vitamin C) by James Lind, a surgeon in the British Royal Navy[3]. However, it was not until the early 1900's that both vitamin discovery and biological characterization of vitamins really started. In fact, the term "vitamine," later shortened to "vitamin" was not coined until 1912 by Casimir Funk.[3] The term was based on the false assumption that all vitamins were "vital amines" (nitrogen containing chemicals in the body) that were necessary for life. Scientists later learned that not all vitamins contain amines, but the term survives to this day.

The first 50 years of the 20th century marked an unprecedented period of investigation of the role of vitamins in disease. Many diseases thought to be caused by bacteria and viruses were in fact vitamin deficiencies.

During the 1800s beriberi was considered to be a contagious disease. Dutch and Japanese physicians noted, however, that consumption by sailors of brown, unpolished rice (with a high thiamine content) decreased the incidence of the disease. In the 1920's two Dutch Scientists chemically isolated and proved deficiency of the vitamin, thiamine, was the cause of beriberi. A similar story was associated with the disease, pellagra.

In the early 1900's, pellagra was rampant in the southern United States. It was believed to be caused by contagious microorganisms. By 1914, Dr. Joseph Goldberger, a physician, proved that pellagra was not a contagion by ingesting body fluid and fecal material from pellagra patients. Apparently, Mrs. Goldberger approved, because she participated in the experiments! The Goldbergers failed to catch pellagra (although it is rumored that it did kill their social life). It was not until the 1930's that the vitamin, niacin, was structurally characterized and found to be the active ingredient in certain foods that prevented or cured pellagra.

And so it went. Throughout the 1920's, 30's and 40's all currently known vitamins were isolated and structurally and biologically characterized. The last to be characterized, vitamin B_{12}, was not described until 1948. During this time, vitamin deficiencies were investigated as the cause or treatments of a wide range of conditions including rickets, pernicious anemia and various types of mental illness, including schizophrenia. Hence, Henry Turkel's attempts to improve the health of persons with Down syndrome in the 1940's via the administration of vitamin and mineral supplements was in keeping with the accepted approach of many biomedical scientists and physicians, during the previous 30 to 40 years. His current characterization as a kook by some sectors of the scientific and medical communities is completely unfounded. Henry Turkel was a man in-step with the scientific and medical thinking of his time. He was also a man ahead of his time. His current critics show their ignorance of the history of nutritional discoveries and their relevance to the reasoning of scientific and medical investigators of the past.

II. Why Henry Turkel was Right About Down Syndrome

Henry Turkel, in his efforts to improve the health of persons with Down syndrome, unknowingly embraced a basic scientific principle that would take decades to become fully appreciated by physicians. It is now axiomatic that **animals and people with different genotypes (different genetic makeup) have different nutritional needs.** [4] Any biologist or agriculturalist deals with this fact of life on a day to day basis caring for animals. Different breeds of animals within the same species have subtle but different nutritional needs. It is not hard to observe this principle in humans in our everyday lives. Have you ever noticed persons of the same height, age and sex as yourself often have no problem maintaining their optimal body weights, in spite of unhealthy dietary habits and lifestyles, while you may have to pay very close attention to dietary intake and exercise to maintain your health? This is due to the fact that you have different genotypes. An extreme example of this principle can be observed in certain Native Americans who consume a modern American/Western European diet. They become morbidly obese and are at very high risk for diabetes, heart disease, cancer and many other diseases.[3]

This principle also applies to persons with Down syndrome. A growing body of both preclinical (laboratory animal research) and clinical research (research with humans) suggests that persons with Down syndrome have different nutritional needs based on fundamental differences in their biochemistry[5] as well as differences in their dietary habits,[6,7] both of which are dictated by in full, or in part, by genotype.

III. What the Critics of Vitamin and Mineral Supplementation Will Not Tell You About Down Syndrome and Nutrition

> "Part of the resistance to megavitamin therapy is based on the idea that an increased intake of a vitamin should be subjected to as thorough testing as a new synthetic drug. This is nonsense; the vitamins are substances to which the human body has long been accustomed, and the toxicities of the water soluble vitamins are known to be low and the side effects few".
>
> Linus Pauling[1]

The use of vitamins to supplement the diet of persons with Down syndrome is constantly criticized by a number of physicians and Down syndrome organizations. Paradoxically, most of the early work linking the cause of diseases to various vitamins was conducted by *physician* investigators. These individuals and organizations are quite vocal and dismissive of any suggestion that dietary supplements can benefit the health of individuals with Down syndrome. Claims are made that there are no scientifically based data to suggest that persons with Down syndrome benefit by vitamin and mineral supplementation at levels greater than found in the typical daily vitamin. Frequently, critics of vitamin supplementation above the published Daily Values cite toxicity as a problem. Most vitamins, including those with the highest potential for toxicity, vitamins A and D, have to be consumed at levels far above those currently being administered to many persons with Down syndrome. Indeed, there are no known toxicity reports in the scientific literature for many of the B vitamins.

> "Neither the nutritional supplements in the doses used, nor the piracetam, appear to be harmful."

Position Statement On Nutritional Intervention In Children With Down Syndrome
(in regards to Targeted Nutritional Intervention – editor)
National Down Syndrome Congress
(http://www.ndsccenter.org/aboutUs/ps_nutrition.asp)

This position of the critics patently ignores a significant body of peer reviewed scientific papers over the last two decades that demonstrate that individuals with Down syndrome are often deficient in many nutrients.[6,8,9,10,11] These individuals are quick to cite scientific papers that show no differences in the needs and effects of vitamin and minerals on Down syndrome persons and the general population. Reconciling conflicting conclusions between studies regarding the same subject are a routine part of the life of a scientist. Scientists consider both the number of papers supporting a given theory as well as the quality of these papers before they formulate a conclusion on the subject. In contrast, the critics of the value of vitamin and mineral supplementation in the management of Down syndrome continually ignore the preponderance of supportive scientific evidence. Additionally, they fail to recognize that these differences in nutritional needs are based on fundamental biochemical differences. Documented differences in the metabolism of persons with Down syndrome include methylation issues,[5] over – expression of the enzyme superoxide dismutase[5] and the excess formation of free radicals.[12] Preclinical studies in Croom's laboratory, with a Down syndrome mouse model, suggest that persons with Down syndrome may not properly metabolize certain amino acids, have excessively high levels of toxic ammonia in their blood and require more energy to absorb nutrients from the intestinal tract.[13,14] Furthermore, persons with Down syndrome absorb more aluminum (Al) than the general population[15] and Down syndrome mouse models indicate they may have higher levels of brain Al.[14] Aluminum accumulation in the brain has been proposed to be one of several variables that cause Alzheimer's disease.[16]

> "The decision by most psychiatrists who do not accept the principles of orthomolecular psychiatry to restrict the intake of vitamins by their patients to certain arbitrary levels, without checking the possible benefit for the patient of an increased intake, cannot be justified".
>
> Orthomolecular therapy: A therapeutic approach to optimizing body functions by optimizing concentrations of substances normally found in the body. Term coined by Linus Pauling-editor.
>
> Linus Pauling[1]

Finally, critics of vitamin supplementation emphasize the lack of evidence for increased cognitive function with nutritional supplementation. This is an important area of research that certainly needs continued and in-depth study. However, little attention has been given to the potential effects of nutrient supplementation on the general health of persons with Down syndrome. Studies in the U.S. (Leichtman, unpublished observations and investigations in progress), Germany[16] and Egypt have documented decreased illness related visits to physicians. Studies in the United States show a significant decrease in upper respiratory, ear and gastrointestinal infections in persons consuming increased levels of vitamin and mineral supplements compared to their peers who did not use similar supplementation. Clinical studies are currently underway at several major universities and medical centers in attempts to understand the biochemical basis of these observations (Shoemaker et al., unpublished observations).

IV. Where are We at and What is The Future of Nutrition Supplementation as a Management Strategy for Down Syndrome ?

The future holds great promise for increased understanding of the unique nutritional needs of persons with Down syndrome. We have come full circle in our thinking of the value of nutritional supplementation in persons with Down syndrome. We have journeyed from a time when vitamin and mineral deficiencies were thought to play a key role in the etiology of Down syndrome, to a time when this approach was considered of no value and back again. Advances in our understanding of a number specific metabolic abnormalities in persons with Down syndrome, as well as awareness of the possible existence of many others, has made the use of nutritional supplements very attractive in the management of this genetic disorder. Until we have a complete understanding of the all the abnormalities in the metabolism of Down syndrome and the variation in occurrence among individuals, administration of broad spectrum vitamin and mineral supplements at elevated (compared to the Federally recommended Daily Values), but non-toxic doses, should be considered prudent. Additionally, any such supplementation should be monitored by physicians and other care givers who have the appropriate training in the health problems associated with Down syndrome as well as a detailed understanding of nutritional biochemistry, physiology and toxicology. Such individuals are not commonly found in the average medical community and must be sought after via the various forums in which information about Down syndrome and its challenges are exchanged.

We will close this brief discussion of the evolution of the nutritional management of Down syndrome by mentioning a recent, exciting discovery. A recent scientific paper published in the prestigious journal, *Nature,*[17] demonstrated that it is possible, in an animal model, to regulate the expression of genes via manipulation of RNA within the cell. This landmark paper could mark the beginning of the development of the ultimate treatment for Down syndrome---the ability to selectively control gene expression on chromosome 21 for enhanced health in trisomic persons. The light at the end of the tunnel for the treatment of persons with Down syndrome may be much closer than we think.

> "I look forward to the day when a Mongolian idiot, treated biochemically, becomes a successful geneticist."
>
> D. J. Kevles
> In the Nature of Eugenics (1985)
>
> Mongolian was an old and inaccurate medical term for persons with Down syndrome. Abandoned by the medical community in 1969 – editor.
>
> Lejeune, Jerome.
> Co-discover of the extra chromosome in Down syndrome

References

1. Orthomolecular Psychiatry: Treatment of Schizophrenia, 1973. D. Hawkins and L. Pauling (eds), W.H. Freeman and Company, San Francisco.

2. Watson, J.D. and F.H. Crick. 1953. *Nature*. 171: 737

3. Whitney, E. N., C. D. Cataldo and S. R. Rolfes. 1998. Understanding Normal and Clinical Nutrition, 5th edition, Wadsworth Publishing Company, London.

4. Simopoulos, A. P. 1999. Nutr. Rev. 57:510

5. Anonymous. 1997. Journal of the American Dietetic Association: 97:189

6. Calvert, S. D., V. M. Vivian, and G. P. Calvert. 1976. J. American Dietetic Association 69: 152-156.

7. Luke, A., M. Sutton, D. A. Schoeller and N. J. M. Roizen. 1996. J. American Dietetic Association 96:1262.

8. Reading, C. M. 1984. Nutr. And Health 3:91

9. Sinet, P. M, J. Neve, A. Nicole and L. Molle. 1984. Acta. Ped. Scand. 73:275

10. Columbo, M.L.,E. Girardo, E. Incarbone, R. Conti, B.M. Ricci and D. Maina. 1989. Minerva Ped. 4:189

11. Sylvester, P.E. 1984. British J. Psych. 145:115

12. Jovanovic, S.V., D. Clements and K. MacLoed. 1998. Free Radical Biol. And Med. 25:1044

13. Cefalu, J., W. J. Croom, E. Eisen, E. Jones, L. Daniel and I. Taylor. 1998. Growth Dev. Aging 62:47

14. Berg, B., J. Croom, J. M. Fernandez, J. W. Spears, E. J. Eisen, I. L. Taylor, L. R. Daniel, B. A. Coles, F. Boeheim and P. J. Mannon. Growth Dev. Aging 64:3

15. Moore, P.B., J. A. Edwardson, I. N. Ferrier, G. A. Taylor, D. Lett, S. P. Tyrer, J. P. Day,S. J. King, and J. S. Lilley. 1997. Biol. Psych 41:488

16. Croom, J. and I. L. Taylor. 2001. J. Inorg. Biochem 87: 51

17. Gelb, J. 2001. Padiatrische Praxis 59: 703

18. Ashrafi, K., F. Y. Chang, J. L. Watts, A. G. Frasers, R. S. Kamath, J. Ahringer and G. Ruvkun. 2003. Nature 421:268

CHAPTER 16:

MANY THANKS

Jenessa just turned 3. She's becoming more independent, more verbal, and even getting quite bossy! She knows what she wants and how to get it. She has plenty of friends, who all love her very much. She touches peoples' lives everywhere she goes. She's taught me, along with the rest of my family, the true meaning of God's grace; His compassion. And what it means to feel pure joy. Children are the purest joy of all.

All children deserve a chance at life. Remember, with or without a disability, all of us are created in the image of God. *All of us!* A child with any syndrome, any disease, any medical impairment, is still a gift from God. Too quickly are these children tossed away due to fear or ignorance. While I realize not every story has a happy ending, I believe that every child deserves a chance. I believe that each child is given to us by God. Who are we to question Him?

A friend of mine told me that she couldn't have brought a disabled child into this world. She is certain that she and her husband wouldn't have had the strength, or desire, to do so. She's really quite insistent about it, and I would never judge her, or anyone else, for their own feelings and choices. However, I pointed out to her that God must have known this about her, because He'd never asked her to do it. He hadn't given her a child that she couldn't handle.

When I first found out about Jenessa, I didn't think I could do it either. But God, in His infinite wisdom, knew that I could. I'm so glad He knew me better than I knew myself.

Another friend of mine desperately needed help. His name is Randy, and he was a painter who spent most of his free time partying. He drank too much, didn't sleep enough, and was addicted to cocaine by the time he was in his mid-thirties. He knew he should straighten up and stop partying, but he was in a rut and having a hard time getting out.

Randy was 37 when he found out he was going to be a father. He'd always loved children, and he needed something in his life to make him more stable. He couldn't have been happier about becoming a dad.

A routine ultrasound during the pregnancy showed some 'funny' shadowing around the baby's heart. Other findings had the doctors thinking about the possibility of Down syndrome, but for whatever reason, no further testing was done.

Whitney was born with Down syndrome. Randy had no understanding of what this meant or what was to come, but vowed to make some major changes in his life. He stopped drinking, stopped doing drugs, and got off his path of self destruction. Whitney needed him.

"Her mother abandoned her," says Randy, "and I knew being a single dad would require every ounce of my energy."

He knew there would be no more time for his partying lifestyle.

Whitney was born with two small holes in her heart. Luckily, by the time she was six months old, they had healed on their own and she did not require surgery. She also had severe respiratory problems, and a very weak immune system. She was prone to infections, colds, and pneumonia. She was hospitalized numerous times, with Randy always by her side.

Doctors found that Whitney lacked the agents which fight off pneumonia. She also lacked the agents that fight the flu, colds, and infections. She had tubes put in her ears because she actually needed them, and hasn't had an ear infection since. She now receives special inoculations in addition to the 'regular' ones that are required, which have helped build back up her immune system. Her health has greatly improved.

Working with the different doctors and helping Whitney get well is all part of what's kept Randy sober.

"Everything I do," says Randy, "I do for her. She has healed me in every way: physically, mentally, emotionally, and spiritually. I am blessed to be her father."

Today Randy owns his own painting company, which allows him

the flexibility to spend more time with his daughter. The two of them rely solely on each other, and are a very special team. Would Randy be where he is today without Whitney? I doubt it. She is his special gift, and *I* believe, given to him by God, to give him a reason to clean up his act. Again, God's infinite wisdom blows me away.

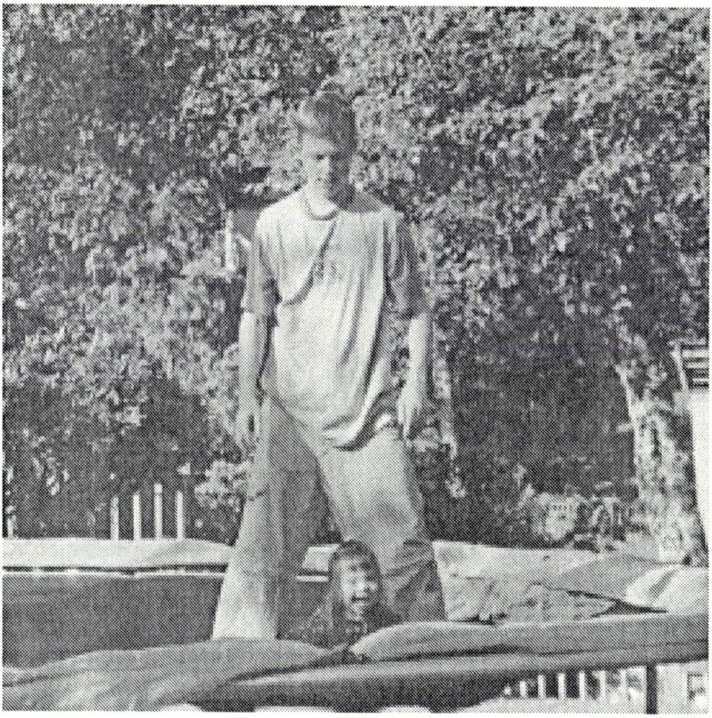

Justin and Jenessa

People often ask me how Justin, Jackie, and Jessi have adapted to having a disabled sister. Justin, who's now 17, adores her. He loves playing rough with her, and she with him. Jackie, now 15, has a very special bond with her. Hers was the first name Jenessa spoke:

"Ackee", she said.

And Jessi, who just turned 7, has no idea what Down syndrome is, or the fact that her sister has it. All Jessi knows is that her sister needs special 'heart batteries' to keep her well. They're the very best of friends.

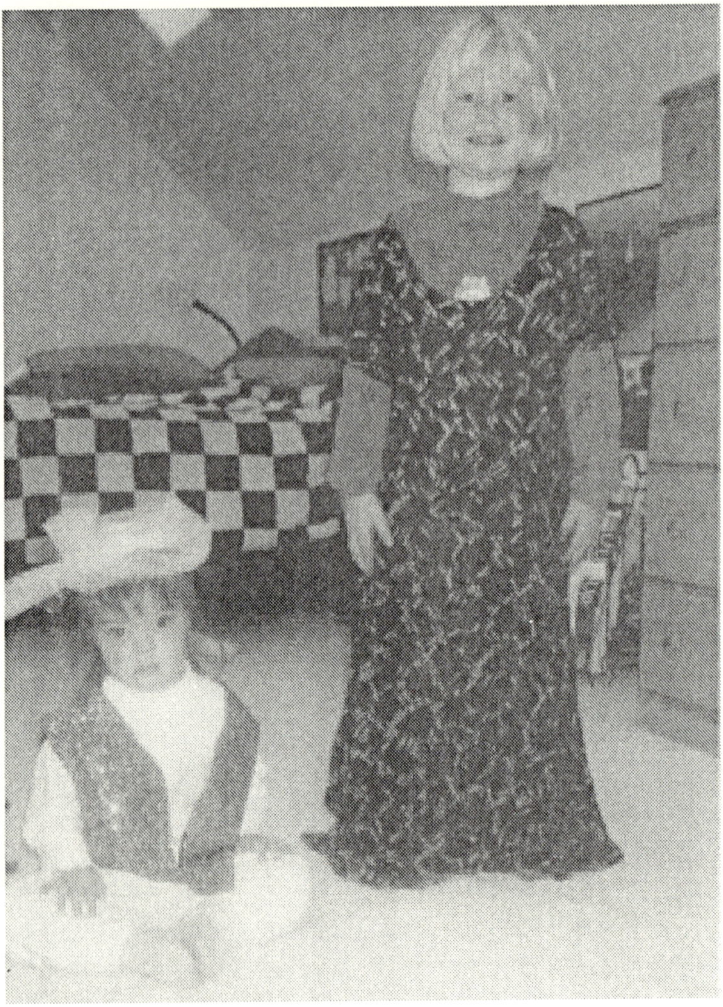

Jessi and Jenessa playing dress-up

Most people have been wonderful to us throughout the first years of Jenessa's life, but I still hear stupid remarks, pretty much on a regular basis. Someone once asked me what was 'wrong' with my child. My answer was simple.

"Nothing."

Just because she's different, doesn't mean she's wrong.

I used to own a children's store, and back when Jenessa was about 16 months old, some lady I had never met was shopping there, and noticed Jenessa was crawling up and down the aisles. She asked me how old she was, and then commented:

"I can't believe she isn't walking yet!"

I said, "No, but she breathes on her own now".

I didn't offer her any further explanations, or excuses, and I didn't pursue the conversation.

Another thing I often hear is how amazed people are that we've survived all that we've been through. They say things like:

"I don't know how you did it." or " I could have never been so strong".

So I ask them what they would do if one of their children were to be involved in a terrible car accident:

"Would you throw your hands up and say no, I can't do this?", "Would you stay away from the hospital because you were too afraid"?

Of course not! The only difference is that we knew in advance about the medical hardships Jenessa would face. Sure we were scared; terrified at times. But we loved Jenessa enough to bring her into this world and weather the storms with her. In return, she has brought us her incredible spirit and boundless love. She has given us so much more than we've given to her. She is truly my miracle from God.

And I thank Him for her every single day. For **all** of my children. I thank Him from the bottom of my soul, mostly for trusting me enough to put them in my care. I am honored beyond words.

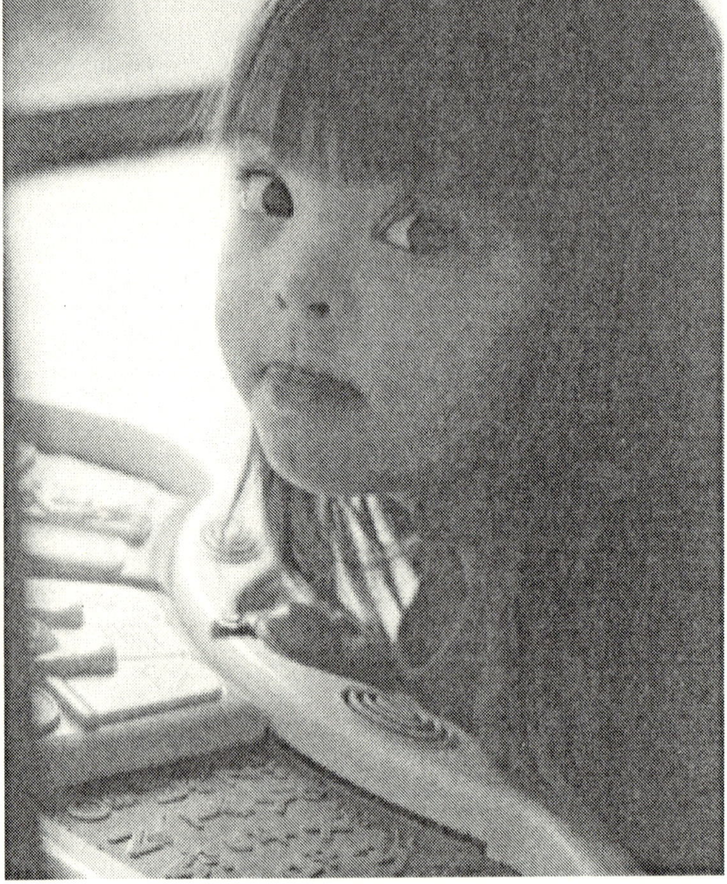

CHAPTER 17:

Tidbits

I'd like to share with you with a short story that was forwarded to me via e-mail a few years ago. It's a fictional story that was written by Dan Anderson, a freelance writer from Iowa. I'm certain it will touch you the same way it's touched me, and so many others.

It is being printed here with his permission:

Something for Stevie

> I try not to be biased, but I had my doubts about hiring Stevie. His placement counselor assured me that he would be a good, reliable busboy, but I'd never had a mentally handicapped employee, and wasn't sure I wanted one. I wasn't sure how my customers would react to Stevie. He was short, a little dumpy, with the smooth facial features and thick-tongued speech of Down syndrome. I wasn't worried about most of my trucker customers, because truckers generally don't care who busses tables as long as the meatloaf platter is good and the pies are homemade. The four-wheeler drivers were the ones who concerned me, the mouthy college kids traveling to school, the yuppie snobs who secretly polish their silverware with their napkins for fear of catching some dreaded truckstop germ, the pairs of white-shirted businessmen on expense accounts who think every truckstop waitress wants to be flirted with. I knew those folks would be uncomfortable around Stevie, so I watched him pretty close the first few weeks. I shouldn't have worried. After the first

week, Stevie had my staff wrapped around his stubby little finger, and within a month my trucker regulars had adopted him as their official truckstop mascot. After that, I really didn't care what the rest of the customers thought of him. He was like a 21-year-old puppy in blue jeans and Nikes, eager to laugh, eager to please, but fierce in his attention to his duties. Every salt and pepper shaker was exactly in place, not a bread crumb or coffee spill visible, when Stevie got done with a table. Our only problem was convincing him to wait to clean up a table until after the customers were finished. He would hover in the background, shifting his weight from one foot to the other, scanning the dining room until a table was empty. Then he would scurry to the empty table and carefully bus the dishes and glasses onto his cart, and meticulously wipe the tabletop with a practiced flourish of his rag. If he thought a nearby customer was watching, his brow would pucker with added concentration. He took pride in doing his job exactly right, and you had to love how hard he tried to please each and every person he met. Over time, we learned that he lived with his mother, a widow, who was disabled after repeated surgeries for cancer. They lived on their Social Security benefits in public housing two miles from the truckstop. Their social worker, who stopped to check on him every so often, admitted that they had "fallen through the cracks." Money was tight, and what I paid him was probably the difference between them being able to live together and Stevie being sent to a group home.

That's why the restaurant was a gloomy place last August, the first morning in three years that Stevie missed work. He was at the Mayo Clinic in Rochester, getting a new valve or something put in his heart. His social worker said that people with Down syndrome often had heart problems at a young age, so this wasn't unexpected, and there was a good chance he would come through the surgery in good shape, and be back at work in a couple months. A ripple of excitement ran through the staff later that morning when word came that he was out of surgery, in recovery, and doing fine. Frannie, my head waitress, let out a war whoop and did a little dance in the aisle when she heard the good news. Big Ben, one of our regular trucker customers, stared at the sight of the fifty-year old, slightly overweight grandmother of four doing a victory shimmy beside his table. Frannie blushed, smoothed her apron and shot Ben a withering look. He grinned.

"Okay, Frannie, what was that all about?" he asked.

"We just got word that Stevie is out of surgery and going to be okay."

"I was wondering where he was. I had a new joke to tell him. What was the surgery about?"

Frannie quickly told Ben and the two other drivers sitting at his booth about Stevie's surgery, then sighed.

"Yeah, I'm glad he's going to be okay," she said, "but I don't know how he and his mom are going to handle all the bills. From what I hear, they're barely getting by as it is."

Big Ben nodded thoughtfully, and Frannie hurried off to wait on the rest of her tables. Since I hadn't had time to round up a busboy to replace Stevie, and really didn't want to replace him, the girls were bussing their own tables, until we decided what to do. After the morning rush, Frannie walked into my office. She had a couple of paper napkins in her hand and a funny look on her face.

"What's up?" I asked.

"I didn't get that table where Big Ben and his friends were sitting cleared off after they left, and Pony Pete and Tony the Tipper were sitting there when I got back to clean it off," she said. "This was folded and tucked under a coffee cup."

She handed the napkin to me, and three $20 bills fell onto my desk when I opened it. On the outside, in big, bold letters, was printed, 'Something for Stevie'.

"Pony Pete asked me what that was all about," she said, "so I told him about Stevie and his mom and everything, and Pete looked at Tony, and Tony looked at Pete, and they ended up giving me this."

She handed me another paper napkin that had, 'Something for Stevie' scrawled on its outside. Two $50 bills were tucked within its folds. Frannie looked at me with wet, shiny eyes, shook her head and said simply, 'Truckers'. That was two months ago. Today is Thanksgiving, the first day Stevie is supposed to be back at work. His placement worker said he's been counting the days until the doctor said he could work, and it didn't matter at all that it was a holiday. He called ten times in the past week, making sure we knew he was coming, fearful that we had forgotten him, or that his job was in jeopardy. I arranged for his mother to bring him to work, met them in the parking lot, and invited them both in to celebrate his first day back. Stevie was thinner, paler, but couldn't stop grinning as he pushed through the doors and headed for the back room where his apron and bussing cart were waiting.

"Hold up there, Stevie, not so fast," I said. I took him and his mother by their arms.

"Work can wait for a minute. To celebrate you coming back, breakfast for you and your mother is on me." I led them toward a large corner booth at the rear of the room. I could feel and hear the rest of the staff following behind as we marched through the dining room. Glancing over my shoulder, I saw booth after booth of grinning truckers empty and join the procession. We stopped in front of the big table. It's surface was covered with coffee cups, saucers, and dinner plates, all sitting slightly crooked on dozens and dozens of folded paper napkins.

"First thing you have to do, Stevie, is clean up this mess," I said.

I tried to sound stern.Stevie looked at me, then at his mother, then pulled out one of the napkins. It had, 'Something for Stevie', printed on the outside. As he picked it up, two $10 bills fell onto the table. Stevie stared at the money, then at all the napkins peeking from beneath the tableware, each with his name printed or scrawled on it. I turned to his mother.

"There's more than $10,000 in cash and checks on that table, all from truckers and trucking companies that heard about your problems. Happy Thanksgiving."

Well, it got real noisy about that time, with everybody hollering and shouting, and there were a few tears as well. But you know what's funny? While everybody else was busy shaking hands and hugging each other, Stevie, with a big, big smile on his face, was busy clearing all the cups and dishes from the table. Best worker I ever hired.

***

First printed in RPM Magazine For Truckers© by Dan

Next is the information I promised you back in chapter one.

...from the American Heart Association

Medical Definitions and Detailed Explanations of Jenessa's heart defects:

Complete Atrioventricular Canal Defect:

> An AV Canal defect is a large hole in the center of the heart. It exists where the wall between the upper chambers joins the wall between the lower chambers. This septal defect involves both upper and lower chambers. Also, the tricuspid and mitral valves that normally separate the heart's upper and lower chambers aren't formed as individual valves. Instead, a single large valve forms that crosses the defect.
>
> The large opening in the center of the heart lets oxygen-rich (red) blood from the heart's left side (blood that's just gone through the lungs) pass into the heart's right side. There, the oxygen-rich blood, along with venous (bluish) blood from the body, is sent back to the lungs. The heart must pump an extra amount of blood and may enlarge. Symptoms may occur at any time from birth to several months of age. Most infants with an AV Canal defect don't grow normally. They also may become undernourished. Because of the large amount of blood flowing to the lungs, high blood pressure may occur there and damage the blood vessels.
>
> In some infants, the common valve between the upper and lower chambers doesn't close properly.

This lets blood leak backward from the heart's lower chambers to the upper ones. This leak, called regurgitation or insufficiency, can occur on the right side, or both sides of the heart. With a valve leak, the heart pumps an extra amount of blood. It becomes overworked and enlarges.

Tetralogy of Fallot:

The Tetralogy of Fallot has four components. The first major one is a *ventricular septal defect.* This is a large hole between the two ventricles that lets venous (bluish) blood pass from the right ventricle to the left one. From there it goes to the aorta and on to the body without passing through the lungs to be refreshed with oxygen.

The second major component of Tetralogy of Fallot is *stenosis,* narrowing at, or just beneath, the pulmonary valve. The narrowing partly blocks the flow of venous blood into the lungs. This varies in severity from child to child. The last two components are: the right ventricle is more muscular than normal; and the aorta lies directly over the ventricular septal defect.

More information on these and other heart defects can be obtained by contacting the American Heart Association,
1-800-242-8721
www.americanheart.org.

****

In closing, I'd like to share with you an essay that was given to me back in the earliest stages of my journey. It was written by Emily

Perl Kingsley, a mother who has a son with Down syndrome. In fact, when her son was born 28 years ago, the doctors suggested that she tell her friends and family that the baby had died in childbirth, and he be institutionalized immediately. Obviously, she didn't choose to do that. Here, with Ms. Kingsley's permission, is her essay:

Welcome To Holland

I am often asked to describe the experience of raising a child with a disability - to try to help people who have not shared that unique experience to understand it, to imagine how it would feel. It's like this......

When you're going to have a baby, it's like planning a fabulous vacation trip - to Italy. You buy a bunch of guide books and make your wonderful plans. The Coliseum. The Michelangelo David. The gondolas in Venice. You may learn some handy phrases in Italian. It's all very exciting.

After months of eager anticipation, the day finally arrives. You pack your bags and off you go. Several hours later, the plane lands. The stewardess comes in and says,

"Welcome to Holland."

"Holland?!?" you say. "What do you mean Holland?? I signed up for Italy! I'm supposed to be in Italy. All my life I've dreamed of going to Italy."

But there's been a change in the flight plan. They've landed in Holland. And there you must stay. The important thing is that they haven't taken you to a horrible, disgusting filthy place, full of pestilence, famine and disease. It's just a different place.

So you must go out and buy new guide books. And you must learn a whole new language. And you will meet a whole new group of people you would never have met.

Holland's just a different place. It's slower-paced than Italy, less flashy than Italy. But after you've been there for a while and you catch your breath, you look around.... and you begin to notice that Holland has windmills....and Holland has tulips. Holland even has Rembrandts.

But everyone you know is busy coming and going from Italy... and they're all bragging about what a wonderful time they had there. And for the rest of your life, you will say

"Yes, that's where I was supposed to go. That's what I had planned."

And the pain of that will never, ever, ever, ever go away... because the loss of that dream is a very, very significant loss.

But... if you spend your life mourning the fact that you didn't get to Italy, you may never be free to enjoy the very special, the very lovely things ...about Holland.

****

Down children truly are specially packaged by God.

What a joy, what a blessing. What an experience!

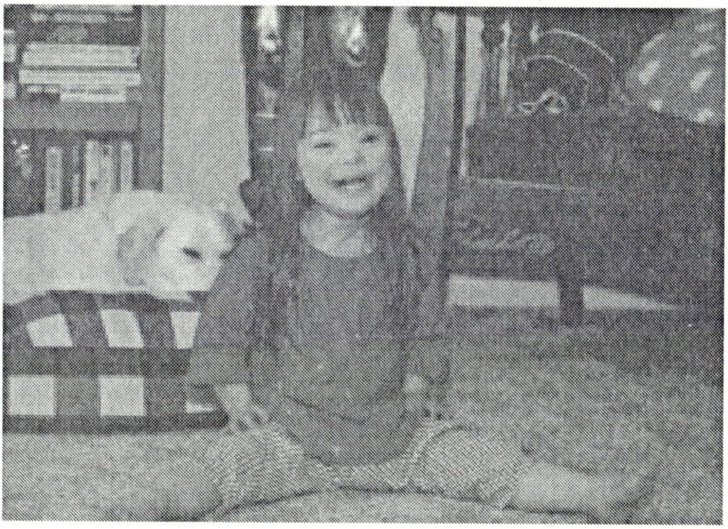

What an incredible gift.

Printed in the United States
119670000lB/127-135